Otolaryngology Surgical Instrument Guide

Otolaryngology Surgical Instrument Guide

Edited by

JUSTIN S. GOLUB, MD
Resident Physician
Research Fellow
Department of Otolaryngology—Head and Neck Surgery
University of Washington
Seattle, WA

and

NICOLE C. SCHMITT, MD
Resident Physician
Research Fellow
Department of Otolaryngology—Head and Neck Surgery
University of Washington
Seattle, WA

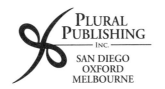

PLURAL
PUBLISHING
— INC. —

SAN DIEGO
OXFORD
MELBOURNE

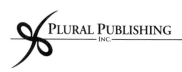

5521 Ruffin Road
San Diego, CA 92123

e-mail: info@pluralpublishing.com
Web site: http://www.pluralpublishing.com

49 Bath Street
Abingdon, Oxfordshire OX14 1EA
United Kingdom

Library of Congress Cataloging-in-Publication Data

Otolaryngology surgical instrument guide / [edited by] Justin S. Golub
and Nicole C. Schmitt.
    p. ; cm.
  Includes bibliographical references and index.
  ISBN-13: 978-1-59756-436-6 (alk. paper)
  ISBN-10: 1-59756-436-2 (alk. paper)
  I. Golub, Justin S. II. Schmitt, Nicole C.
  [DNLM: 1. Otorhinolaryngologic Surgical Procedures—instrumenta-
tion. 2. Reconstructive Surgical Procedures—instrumentation. WV 26]

  617.952—dc23
                        2011041071

Contents

Preface

Justin S. Golub

I remember my disbelief at the senior resident's response during my medical school surgical clerkship.

"You just figure it out over time, pick it up piece by piece," he explained after a shrug.

"Really? You mean you don't study it in a book? You can't look it up?" I asked, astonished.

"No, there are no books. It just comes, somehow."

My questioning regarded a long-term fascination of mine: surgical instrumentation. Throughout my professional education, it has bewildered me that there is no systematic way to study the tools essential to our operative endeavors. These tools affect our movements, decisions, and intentions. The choice of what to use and how to use it distinguishes a skillful surgeon. Yet within surgical disciplines, there are no resources to systematically learn and study instruments.

Heeding the words of my former resident, I entered my own residency anticipating that somehow, perhaps through osmosis, the names and specific functions of instruments would simply come to me. In a few cases they did. The omnipresent DeBakey forceps, for example, quickly became a familiar friend. But for the majority of instruments, becoming acquainted was a great challenge.

One hurdle was that different attendings used different instruments, even for the same operation. I would become accustomed to employing the Cottle for a particular maneuver, only to be scolded months later and told that a Freer was the tool to use. Even more exasperating was that different attendings used different nicknames for the same instrument. And on traveling to a different hospital, the entire tray composition would change.

I found myself never knowing precisely what to ask for, despite knowing the next step in the procedure. "Hemostat," I would say, only to be met with a blank stare by the scrub technician. After a pause, she would suggest a Crile. In an attempt to accelerate the learning curve, I would ask questions. "How is a Crile different from a Jake, or a Kelly from a Pean?" But the fast-paced OR environment was often not conducive to interrogations about instrument naming.

Even if I did receive direct training on instrumentation during a case, it certainly was not the ideal environment for studying. In particular, there was no way to take notes when scrubbed in. Between cases (a frenetic scramble to write orders, dictate, transfer the patient, and meet the next), the timing was no better.

One could point to instrument catalogs of major manufacturers. However, these "telephone books" of photos and names are not designed in an accessible format. Most critically, they lack an explanation on how and why to use particular instruments. Step-by-step assembly instructions of complex yet lifesaving devices, such as a pediatric bronchoscope for a foreign body removal, cannot be found anywhere. Ironically, it is the faultlessly unprepared junior resident with no pediatrics experience who may arrive at the operating room first in the middle of the night charged with the task of setup.

Over the years, I did somehow grow comfortable with a basic core of instruments. My tone when requesting tools evolved from questioning to decisive requesting. It became natural and routine. Yet when a medical student would occasionally scrub in on a case with me, I would find myself struggling to explain how on earth I ever learned the names of so many instruments.

These experiences were the inspiration behind *Otolaryngology Surgical Instrument Guide*. My coeditor, Nikki Schmitt, and I resolved to create a trainee-friendly guidebook to the essential tools we spend countless hours with, the tools that affect our decisions and physical motions. They are quite literally the connection between surgeon and patient.

We reasoned that if residents were comfortable with the appearance, terminology, and usage of major surgical instruments before cases, their comfort level in the operating room would rise. In turn, they could focus on learning the steps of the operation rather than the identity of the unfamiliar object that was just placed in their hand.

The first hurdle was obtaining images. A comprehensive guide would have to include subspecialty instruments sold through numerous vendors; obtaining copyright permissions would be a nightmare. We decided early on to photograph instruments ourselves. With a little personal photojournalism experience and a heap of optimism we embarked on the task.

One sunny call-free morning, we stormed into the operating room and set up a studio. I remember that first experience quite well: we were armed with a shiny Macintosh laptop, two enormous bags of photographic equipment (including items borrowed from some very generous colleagues), and a giant sheet of white oak tag. The setup was every bit as intricate and time consuming as for an actual OR case.

We draped the area, set up the tripod, flash, and diffuser, taped down cables, connected the camera to the computer, and set up an instrument assembly line. As with all big projects, we underestimated the work required. We anticipated four shoots to capture all needed instruments. In the end, the project required nine.

It turns out that reflective metallic instruments are incredibly difficult to photograph. The light from the flash bounces straight back, "blowing out" the highlights and obscuring the precious contrast details. With meticulous adjustment of the flashes and instrument angles, we were able to suppress this lighting side effect in most cases. The most time-consuming part of the photographic effort was editing, retouching, and matching each photo to the text. We took several thousand photographs in total, although the majority of those did not make the cut.

The more we photographed, the more the work seemed to transcend into art. Staring at the smooth, scintillating metallic instruments with their sharp shadows and rich highlights became beautiful, a word not typically associated with blood-covered scissors and forceps. This was one of the many gratifying aspects of the journey.

We hope that *Otolaryngology Surgical Instrument Guide* will prove insightful to the hundreds of medical students and otolaryngology residents who study our surgical field each year. In broader context, the guide might also help non-familiar operating room personnel become more facile with our highly specialized (or in some cases, frankly, obscure) instruments. This would undoubtedly have a direct positive impact on operating surgeons and their patients.

Preface

Nicole C. Schmitt

During the first year of clinical training in otolaryngology, the resident is exposed to a vast amount of new information. Included in the list of new material to learn are hundreds of surgical instruments, which are at first frustratingly unfamiliar. How does one select the appropriate laryngoscope among the several scopes in the bronchoscopy cart? What is a whirlybird? A Buckingham mirror? How do I set up for an emergent airway case in the middle of the night? Where can I read about these things?

I eventually learned the answers to these instrumentation questions through experience, but I was quite surprised to find that the only existing resources for referencing surgical instruments in our field were manufacturers' instrument catalogs, each of which contained a potpourri of different instruments but virtually no information about how each instrument is used. There were several books about general surgical instrumentation intended for scrub personnel; I purchased one of them and was dismayed to find that the section on airway instruments contained a grand total of two instruments.

I realized that in order to have a good reference on surgical instruments for otolaryngology, someone from our field would have to create it. To test feasibility, I brought my camera to the operating room and tried to photograph a tray of instruments. Taking good photographs indoors without adequate lighting proved difficult. I presented the idea of a surgical instrument guide to a handful of residents and faculty from our department as a practice-based learning project. Did anyone else think this would be useful? Did anyone have any photography tips? The consensus was that although it would be useful for trainees to have a comprehensive, photographic guide of surgical instrumentation, compiling it from scratch and publishing it would be a huge and perhaps unrealistic undertaking. I resigned myself to getting photographs from the Internet to make an "unofficial" instrument guide to share with my fellow residents.

My future coeditor, Justin Golub, was away that day enjoying the ski slopes on a long-awaited vacation. Several months later he queried his fellow residents: Did anyone think it would be useful to have a photographic guide of commonly used surgical instruments for otolaryngology?

What were the chances that a fellow resident would independently develop the same idea, and that he would be a photographer to boot? We were now a team with a shared goal. We did a test shoot with a tray of instruments and obtained some very decent photographs. With renewed enthusiasm, we decided to embark on what would become over a year of photographing, measuring, and researching instruments. We recruited residents and faculty to write about the instruments related to their subspecialties of interest. We edited, cross-referenced, rephotographed, and re-edited.

The result is the first book on surgical instrumentation specifically intended for otolaryngology — head and neck surgeons and other staff who work frequently in our field. While fairly comprehensive, our specialty is amazingly broad, and no single book can possibly contain every instrument that we use. There are also some institutional biases, as we logistically could only photograph instruments that our affiliated institutions possess. I am also sure that some of the nicknames are used more prominently here than elsewhere. Those caveats aside, we hope that this book will be informative. Whether you are a medical student interested in otolaryngology, an otolaryngology resident, a scrub technician who has recently begun scrubbing in for otolaryngology cases, or a senior faculty member trying to remember the name of that one instrument you might have used ten years ago, we are delighted to share with you our enthusiasm for these wonderful tools that enhance our ability to care for patients.

Instrument Key

Basic terminology for surgical instrumentation, including instrument components, is illustrated and defined below. This is not intended to be comprehensive, but rather a framework of vocabulary that will make the remainder of this book easily understandable.

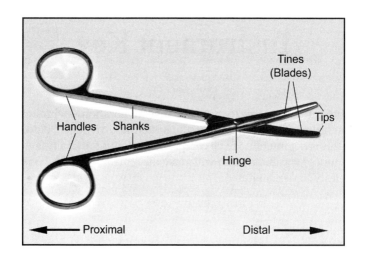

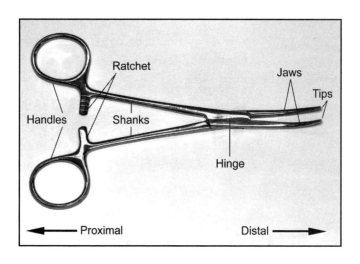

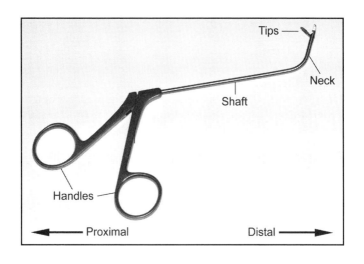

Tips

Neck

Shaft

Handles

Proximal   Distal

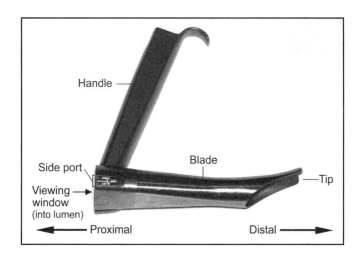

Handle

Side port

Viewing
window
(into lumen)

Blade

Tip

Proximal   Distal

Blade   Any flat, wide structure. May be sharp and used for cutting (eg, #15 blade), or dull and used for retracting (eg, blades of a nasal speculum).

Distal   Part of the instrument that is farther from the surgeon's hand.

Double-action   A mechanism that includes multiple hinges instead of one, greatly increasing power at the instrument jaws when squeezing the handles (eg, double-action rongeur).

Flange   A protruding rim or collar, often used to hold an object in place or facilitate attachment to another object (eg, flange of a tracheotomy tube).

Forceps   General term for any instrument that may be used to compress or grasp tissue. Includes ring-handled instruments (which often contain a ratcheting clamp mechanism) or instruments that resemble "tweezers."

Handle   Part of an instrument that the surgeon holds.

Hemostat   General term for any instrument that may stop bleeding by compressing blood vessels. Usually pertains to so-called hemostatic forceps, which contain a ratcheting clamp mechanism.

Hinge   Movable joint, such as the screwlike hinge immediately proximal to scissor tines.

Jaws   Part of an instrument used for grasping another structure, such as the jaws of a needle driver or the jaws of a clamp.

Knurled   A pattern of fine ridges created on the surface of metal instruments to aid in gripping.

Neck   Component of an instrument that is located between the shaft and the tip. To be present, must be structurally distinct from the shaft. Often is angled or curved.

Proximal   Part of instrument that is closer to the surgeon's hand.

Rasp   Short for raspatory. An instrument used for scraping or coarsely filing bone.

Ratchet   Ridged structure often immediately distal to ring handles. Enables instruments to act as clamps via a locking mechanism.

Ring-handled   Describes an instrument with handles that include finger rings (eg, in scissors).

Scope   General term for any instrument used to look into body cavities via a natural or surgically created orifice. May include optical devices such as rigid telescopes (term used synonymously with rigid endoscopes) or nonoptical hollow metal devices such as rigid laryngoscopes, rigid broncho-scopes, and rigid esophagoscopes. Flexible scopes, which are used less commonly in the operating room, are beyond the scope of this book.

Shaft   Central rodlike component of an instrument.

Shank   Central rodlike component of a ring-handled instru-ment (eg, shanks of scissors or clamps).

Tine   A slender pronglike structure (eg, tines of scissors).

Tip   The most distal aspect of an instrument.

Acknowledgments

We greatly appreciate the help of the following individuals for their time and expertise: Jacquelyn Walker, Melissa Marshburn, Maria Cudejkova, Pam Auxier, Greg Kinzel, Robert Browne, Leah Norton, Sheri Kinley, Lawrence Golub, DDS, and the operating room and instrument processing staff at the University of Washington Medical Center, Seattle Children's Hospital, and Harborview Medical Center.

We also thank Prabhat Bhama, MD, and Amit Bhrany, MD, for lending select photographic tools.

Contributing Authors

Karthik Balakrishnan, MD, MPH
Resident Physician
Department of Otolaryngology — Head and Neck Surgery
University of Washington
Seattle, Washington
Chapter 5

Prabhat K. Bhama, MD
Resident Physician
Department of Otolaryngology — Head and Neck Surgery
University of Washington
Seattle, Washington
Chapter 6

Amit D. Bhrany, MD
Assistant Professor
Department of Otolaryngology — Head and Neck Surgery
University of Washington
Seattle, Washington
Chapter 6

Greg E. Davis, MD, MPH
Assistant Professor
Department of Otolaryngology — Head and Neck Surgery
University of Washington
Seattle, Washington
Chapter 3

Justin S. Golub, MD
Resident Physician
Department of Otolaryngology — Head and Neck Surgery

University of Washington
Seattle, Washington
Chapter 2

Jae H. Lim, MD, PhD
Resident Physician
Department of Otolaryngology—Head and Neck Surgery
University of Washington
Seattle, Washington
Chapter 3

Jack J. Liu, MD
Resident Physician
Department of Otolaryngology—Head and Neck Surgery
University of Washington
Seattle, Washington
Chapter 4

Eduardo Mendez, MD, MS, FACS
Assistant Professor
Department of Otolaryngology—Head and Neck Surgery
University of Washington
Assistant Member
Clinical Research Division
Fred Hutchinson Cancer Research Center
Seattle, Washington
Chapter 1

Tanya K. Meyer, MD
Assistant Professor
Department of Otolaryngology—Head and Neck Surgery
University of Washington
Seattle, Washington
Chapter 4

Kris S. Moe, MD, FACS
Associate Professor
Chief, Division of Facial Plastic Surgery
Department of Otolaryngology—Head and Neck Surgery

University of Washington
Seattle, Washington
Chapter 6

Jay T. Rubinstein, MD, PhD
Professor and Director
Virginia Merrill Bloedel Hearing Research Center
Department of Otolaryngology—Head and Neck Surgery
University of Washington
Seattle, Washington
Chapter 2

Nicole C. Schmitt, MD
Resident Physician
Department of Otolaryngology—Head and Neck Surgery
University of Washington
Seattle, Washington
Chapter 1

Arun Sharma, MD, MS
Resident Physician
Department of Otolaryngology—Head and Neck Surgery
University of Washington
Seattle, Washington
Chapter 4

Kathleen C. Y. Sie, MD
Professor
Department of Otolaryngology—Head and Neck Surgery
University of Washington
Seattle Children's Hospital
Seattle, Washington
Chapter 2 and 5

To my wife, Katrina, for her infinite patience and support. And to my mother, Carol, my father, Larry, and my sister, Danielle, for their kindness and encouragement.

Justin S. Golub

To my husband, Renaud, for his unwavering support and patience, and to my mother, Debbie, whose talent never ceases to amaze and inspire me.

Nicole C. Schmitt

CHAPTER

Head and Neck Surgery

Nicole C. Schmitt and Eduardo Mendez

CONTENTS

Lahey Forceps
Vessel Clamps

Scissors
Mayo Scissors (Straight)
Mayo Scissors (Curved)
Metzenbaum Scissors
Tenotomy Scissors
Iris Scissors (Curved)
Iris Scissors (Straight)

Retractors
Malleable Retractor
Cummings Retractor
Richardson Retractor
Deaver Retractor
Senn Retractor
Ragnell Retractor
Volkmann Rake Retractor
Green Retractor
Army-Navy Retractor
Langenbeck Retractor
Weider Retractor
University of Minnesota Retractor
Bite Block
Weitlaner Self-Retaining Retractor
Articulating Weitlaner Self-Retaining Retractor
Double-Pronged Hook
Double-Pronged Hook, Fine
Single-Pronged Hook

General and Miscellaneous Instruments
Scalpel Handle #3
Scalpel Handle #7
Scalpel Blades #10, #11, #15
Needle Driver
Vascular Clip Applier
Wire Cutters

Towel Clamp, Penetrating
Towel Clamp, Nonpenetrating
Bipolar Cautery Forceps
Bovie Electrocautery
Suction Bovie Electrocautery
Yankauer Suction
Frazier Suction
Baron Suction
McCabe Facial Nerve Dissector

Instruments for Robotic Surgery

Feyh-Kastenbauer Laryngopharyngoscope (With Attachments)
Da Vinci Robot EndoWrist Instruments
Kuppersmith Robotic Thyroidectomy Retractor Set

Forceps

Bayonet Forceps

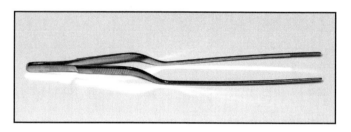

Aliases and Nicknames: Bayonets

Uses: Primarily used for grasping objects (inserting or removing) in the nasal cavity. The double bend is designed so that the surgeon's hand is lower than the grasped object to prevent the surgeon's hand from obstructing the view of the object.

Description: Forceps with a double bend midway down the shaft, so that the axis of the tines sits 1 to 2 cm higher than the handle.

Dimensions: ~21 cm long (varies)

DeBakey Forceps

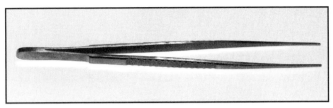

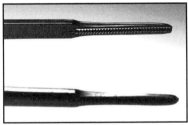

Aliases and Nicknames: DeBakeys

Uses: Handling/grasping tissue other than skin. Often used to atraumatically grasp bleeding vessels (can then touch the forceps with a Bovie to cauterize).

Description: Long forceps with numerous fine teeth arranged in a longitudinal pattern to allow atraumatic gripping.

Dimensions: ~15–19 cm long (varies)

Tips and Pitfalls: Avoid using on skin, which can be crushed by DeBakey forceps; use forceps with sharp teeth at the very tip (eg, Adson forceps) instead.

Adson Forceps

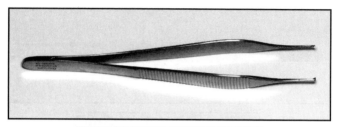

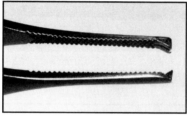

Aliases and Nicknames: Adson pickups, Adsons

Uses: Grasping skin and other tissues that should not be crushed.

Description: Relatively short forceps with three prominent teeth that interlock. Adsons without teeth also exist for delicate handling of tissue other than skin.

Dimensions: ~12–15 cm long (varies)

Tips and Pitfalls: Use them routinely to close skin incisions. Handle tissue carefully with these forceps; although they won't usually crush skin, they can pierce holes or tear delicate skin. For more delicate skin work, use the finer Bishop-Harmon forceps (see p. 299).

Adson-Brown Forceps

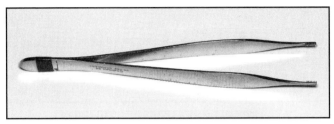

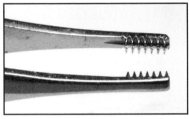

Aliases and Nicknames: Adson-Brown pickups, Browns, Brown-Adson, Adson-Browns

Uses: Gripping tissue.

Description: Similar to Adson forceps, but with two pairs of ~7 interlocking teeth on each tine for improved gripping.

Dimensions: ~12–15 cm long (varies)

Tips and Pitfalls: Avoid using extensively on skin and cartilage, as the teeth can crush these tissues.

Gerald Forceps (With or Without Teeth)

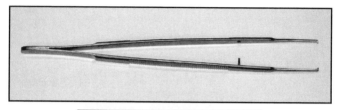

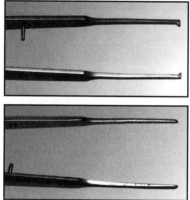

Aliases and Nicknames: Geralds

Uses: Grasping delicate tissue that should not be crushed.

Description: Long forceps with an abrupt narrowing near the distal sixth of the instrument. Tips can be with teeth (second image above) or serrated (third image above).

Dimensions: ~18 cm long

Tips and Pitfalls: Use Geralds with teeth carefully to avoid traumatizing tissue.

Jacobson Forceps

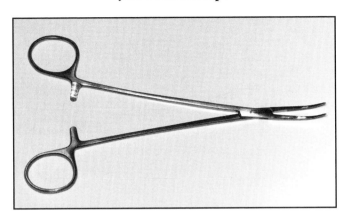

Aliases and Nicknames: Jake forceps, Jake clamp, Jake, fine tonsil

Uses: Delicate dissection and clamping of blood vessels.

Description: Long, thin, ring-handled forceps with ratcheting clamp mechanism and fine tines.

Dimensions: ~19 cm long (varies)

Tips and Pitfalls: When clamping a vessel, use a Jake on either side of the area to be cut and ligated, with the curves of the two forceps facing each other. Jake tips are very fine; in situations where delicate tissue should not be punctured, consider using forceps with larger tips for more blunt dissection. Some surgeons use Jakes only for dissection and never for clamping tissue to avoid damaging the tips.

Mosquito Forceps

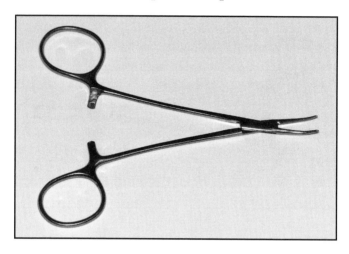

Aliases and Nicknames: Mosquito, hemostat, snap, tag, Hartman mosquito (slightly smaller), Halstead mosquito (slightly larger)

Uses: Holding tissue or clamping blood vessels. Also frequently used to hold (tag) sutures and other materials so that they are not lost or pulled out.

Description: Small, delicate, ring-handled forceps with ratcheting clamp mechanism and fine, curved (as pictured) or straight tips with transverse grooves for grasping.

Dimensions: 9–12 cm long

Kelly Hemostatic Forceps

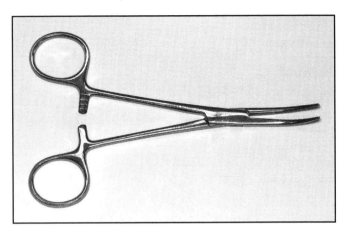

Aliases and Nicknames: Kelly, Kelly clamp, curved (or straight) Kelly

Uses: Clamping larger blood vessels, holding tissue, and blunt dissection.

Description: Ring-handled forceps with ratcheting clamp mechanism and curved (as pictured above) or straight tips with transverse grooves for grasping. Transverse grooves do not extend all the way proximally to the hinge.

Dimensions: 12–14 cm long (varies)

Tips and Pitfalls: Similar forceps include the following:

- *Crile forceps* are a similar design. In Crile forceps, the transverse grooves extend the full length from the tip to the hinge.
- *Schnidt (tonsil) forceps* have a longer handle (19 cm instrument length). One of the ring handles is often incomplete. During tonsillectomy, a sponge ball is placed in the jaws of the Schnidt forceps, and this is used to tamponade bleeding from the tonsillar fossa.

Rochester-Pean Hemostatic Forceps

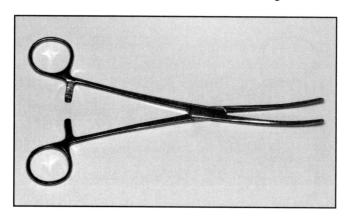

Uses: Clamping tissue and large vessels.

Description: Large ring-handled forceps with ratcheting clamp mechanism and curved (as pictured) or straight tips with deep transverse grooves for grasping.

Dimensions: 23 cm long

Right Angle Forceps

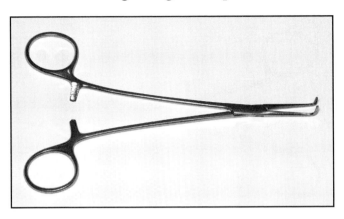

Aliases and Nicknames: Right angle

Uses: Clamping in general; can be particularly useful for reaching around corners to grasp or clamp objects or tissue.

Description: Long ring-handled forceps with ratcheting clamp mechanism and fine tines at a 90° angle to the axis of the rest of the instrument. Tips of tines sometimes contain fine transverse grooves for gripping.

Dimensions: 18 cm long

Kocher Forceps

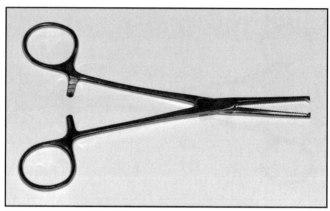

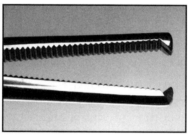

Aliases and Nicknames: Kocher, Kocher clamp

Uses: Used to firmly grip relatively large areas of tissue or objects (eg, suction tubing).

Description: Ring-handled forceps with ratcheting clamp mechanism and heavy tips that have deep transverse grooves and large interlocking teeth at the distal end. Tips can be straight (as pictured) or curved.

Dimensions: 16 cm long

Allis Tissue Forceps

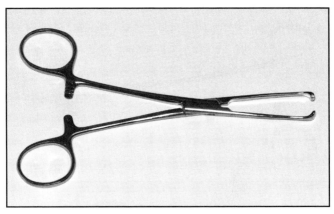

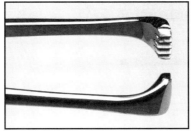

Aliases and Nicknames: Allis, curved Allis, tonsil tenaculum (curved version)

Uses: Grasping tissue (eg, tonsils) for retraction while minimizing trauma.

Description: Ring-handled forceps with ratcheting clamp mechanism and distal ends that curve toward each other, with 5 pairs of interlocking teeth. Tips can be straight (as pictured) or curved.

Dimensions: 16 cm long

Tips and Pitfalls: Avoid excessive clamping/pulling of tissue with the Allis, which can be traumatic.

Babcock Tissue Forceps

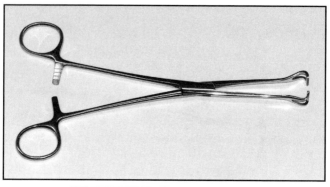

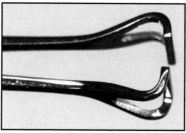

Aliases and Nicknames: Babcock

Uses: Grasping tissue (eg, wall of a cyst) for retraction while minimizing trauma.

Description: Ring-handled forceps with ratcheting clamp mechanism and looped distal ends that curve toward each other.

Dimensions: ~16 cm long

Lahey Forceps

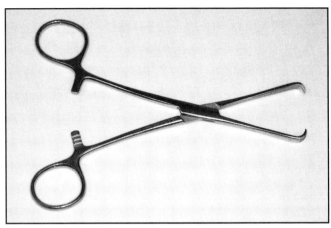

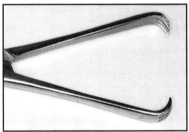

Aliases and Nicknames: Lahey

Uses: Grasping and retracting.

Description: Ring-handled forceps with ratcheting clamp mechanism and distal ends that curve toward each other. Tips contain multiple pairs of large, sharp, interlocking teeth. Region near the tip may be straight (as pictured) or curved. Teeth are sharper and more prominent than on Allis forceps.

Dimensions: 16 cm long

Tips and Pitfalls: Strong retraction with the Lahey forceps can lead to avulsion or damage of delicate tissues or cartilage. Sharp teeth may also damage tissue.

Vessel Clamps

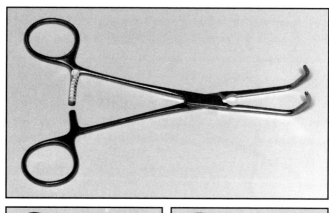

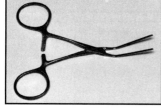
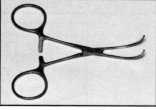

Uses: Atraumatic temporary occlusion of blood vessels in situations where the vessels will not be ligated (eg, when anastomosing a vein in an end-to-side fashion to the internal jugular vein).

Description: Ring-handled ratcheting clamp with upward-curving or upward-bent tines. (Three variations are displayed above.) Tines may contain a ridged medial surface reminiscent of DeBakey forceps (see p. 5).

Dimensions: ~11–16 cm long (varies)

Scissors

Mayo Scissors (Straight)

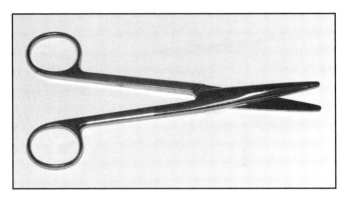

Aliases and Nicknames: Mayo, Mayos, heavy Mayos, heavy scissors, suture scissors

Uses: Multipurpose scissors used for cutting suture, dressings, and other nondelicate material. Also used for large tissue cuts.

Description: Large, heavy scissors with blades that are moderately sharp. Tips are blunt.

Dimensions: 17 cm long

Mayo Scissors (Curved)

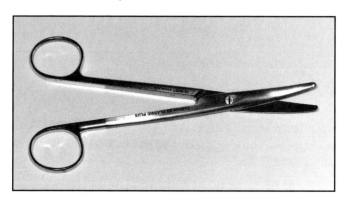

Aliases and Nicknames: Curved Mayo, curved Mayos

Uses: Similar to straight Mayo scissors. Also frequently used in tracheotomy procedures. After a horizontal cut is made in the trachea with a scalpel, these are used to make vertical cuts in the trachea for creation of a tracheal window or Bjork flap.

Description: Large, heavy scissors with curved blades that are moderately sharp. Tips are blunt.

Dimensions: 17 cm long

Metzenbaum Scissors

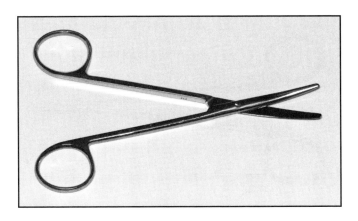

Aliases and Nicknames: Metz, curved Metz

Uses: Cutting or dissecting delicate tissues.

Description: Long, thin, fine scissors of various sizes, with relatively short blades compared with the length of the shanks. Blades are sharp for fine cutting and dissecting, and usually are curved. Tips are blunt.

Dimensions: ~14–18 cm long (varies)

Tenotomy Scissors

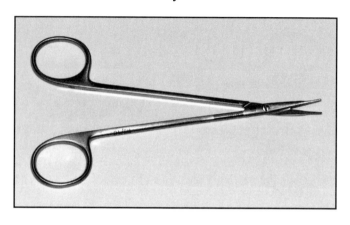

Aliases and Nicknames: Tenotomy

Uses: Delicate dissection.

Description: Fine scissors with short, sharp blades. Tips narrow out quickly and then more gradually to create a "duck bill" appearance. The distal tips are finer than in Metzenbaum scissors, but blunt compared to those of iris scissors (see next entry).

Dimensions: ~15 cm long (varies)

Iris Scissors (Curved)

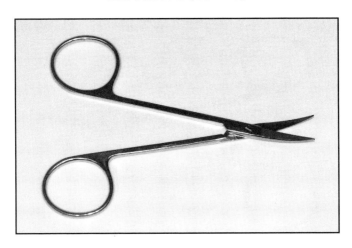

Aliases and Nicknames: Curved irises, suture scissors (when cutting fine suture)

Uses: Used for a variety of purposes, from cutting fine suture or dressing materials to fine dissection and cutting of tissue.

Description: Short, fine scissors with fine, sharp, curved blades. Tips are sharp.

Dimensions: 11 cm long

Iris Scissors (Straight)

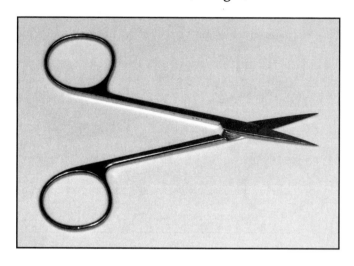

Aliases and Nicknames: Irises, suture scissors (when cutting fine suture)

Uses: Used for a variety of purposes, from cutting fine suture or dressing materials to fine dissection and cutting of tissue. Used less frequently for dissection than curved iris scissors.

Description: Short, fine scissors with fine, sharp, straight blades. Tips are sharp.

Dimensions: 11 cm long

Note: For palate scissors, see pp. 222–223. For other specialized scissors, see pp. 261–267.

Retractors

Malleable Retractor

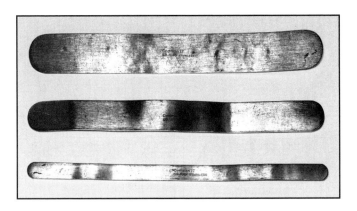

Aliases and Nicknames: Malleable

Uses: Useful for retracting under a variety of circumstances. Can be bent to the appropriate curvature.

Description: Long, thin, and flat metal retractor with rounded corners that can be bent to the desired curvature.

Dimensions: ~17 cm long, various widths

Tips and Pitfalls: Malleable instruments can wear out if bent frequently, after which they need to be replaced. Bending is performed by hand.

Cummings Retractor

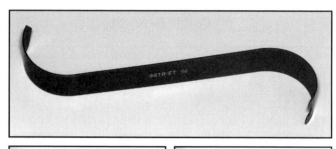

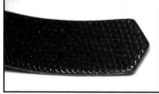
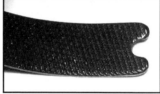

Aliases and Nicknames: Cummings

Uses: Retracting in a variety of situations, including neck dissections.

Description: Long, thin S-shaped metal retractor with two opposing curves. One end has a triangular point and one end has a U-shaped groove. The concave sides of the curved ends have a knurled texture.

Dimensions: 14–19 cm long (varies)

Tips and Pitfalls: Hands may fatigue when retracting with this instrument for long periods of time due to lack of an ergonomic handle.

Richardson Retractor

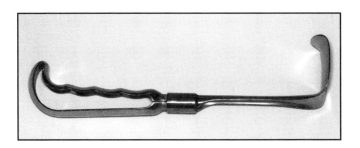

Aliases and Nicknames: Rich

Uses: Retracting large amounts of tissue. Used for neck surgery, free flap reconstruction, and other large surgical fields.

Description: Large, handled retractor with a scooped lip. The main portion of the lip is at a 90° angle with the remainder of the instrument.

Dimensions: 25 cm long (varies)

Deaver Retractor

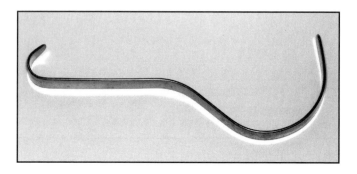

Aliases and Nicknames: Deaver

Uses: Retracting large amounts of tissue.

Description: Large C-shaped retracting end that occupies the distal half of the instrument.

Dimensions: Varies

Senn Retractor

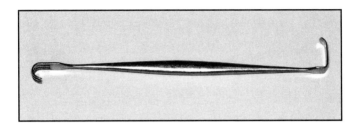

Aliases and Nicknames: Senn

Uses: One of the most commonly used retractors in head and neck surgery. Employed in tracheotomy, thyroid surgery, and a variety of other neck surgeries with small or moderate sized fields.

Description: Fine retractor with C-shaped, rakelike lip on one end with either sharp or blunt teeth. The other end contains a blunt lip at a 90° angle to the shaft with a gentle concavity at the most distal tip.

Dimensions: 16 cm long

Tips and Pitfalls: Beware of sharp injuries to the hand of the person retracting, which can occur easily while using the blunt end for retraction and holding the sharp rake end.

Ragnell Retractor

See p. 258.

Volkmann Rake Retractor

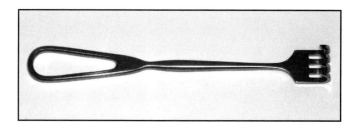

Aliases and Nicknames: Rake

Uses: Retracting large areas of tissue (eg, sternocleidomas-toid and other large muscles).

Description: Long retractor with sharp, rakelike end.

Dimensions: 23 cm long

Green Retractor

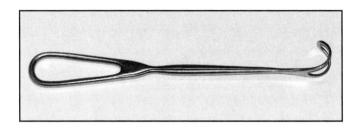

Aliases and Nicknames: Green goiter retractor

Uses: Retracting muscle or soft tissue during thyroidectomy and other neck procedures.

Description: Long handled retractor with curved, looped distal end.

Dimensions: ~23 cm long

Army-Navy Retractor

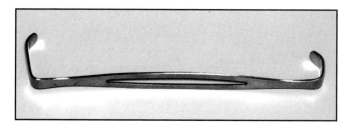

Aliases and Nicknames: Army-Navy, U.S. Army retractor

Uses: Commonly used retractor in tracheotomy and other neck surgeries. The shorter end can be used for retracting more shallow tissues, whereas the longer end can be used for deeper retraction as the surgery progresses.

Description: Long, thin retractor with two J-shaped ends, one longer than the other.

Dimensions: 22 cm long

Langenbeck Retractor

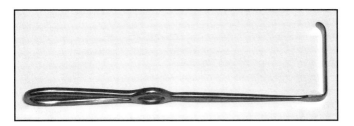

Aliases and Nicknames: Langenbeck

Uses: Used for retracting in deep tissues, including the oral cavity/cheek.

Description: Long, handled retractor with a flat retracting lip that is at a 90° angle to the remainder of the instrument. The most distal tip has a gentle concavity.

Dimensions: 23 cm long, retracting lip varies in width and length

Weider Retractor

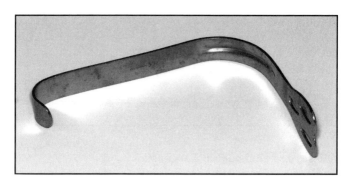

Aliases and Nicknames: Sweetheart retraction, Weider tongue depressor

Uses: Commonly used to retract the tongue inferiorly for better visualization of the oral cavity/oropharynx. Can also be used to retract the cheek.

Description: Ridged, heart-shaped, flat retracting tip with three teardrop-shaped holes. 90° bends in the neck and proximal handle. (Handle depicted on the left in the image above.)

Dimensions: 13 cm long (long axis)

University of Minnesota Retractor

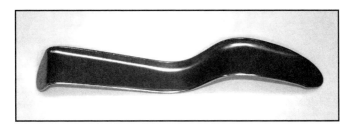

Aliases and Nicknames: Minnesota, cheek retractor

Uses: Retracting the cheek and lips.

Description: Flat, gently curved, rounded tip for retracting. Contains a bayonet-style double bend that offsets the tip from the handle. Lateral edges are bent superiorly except at the distal-most and proximal-most ends. (Handle depicted on the left in the image above.)

Dimensions: 14 cm long

Bite Block

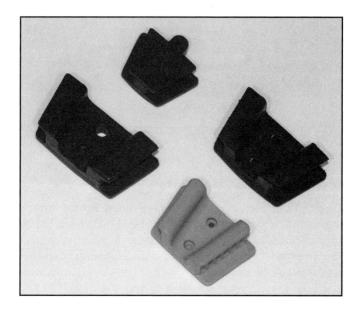

Uses: Used to hold the maxillary and mandibular teeth apart to facilitate operating in the oral cavity.

Description: Rubber trapezoid-shaped blocks with grooves on the sides designed to accommodate the teeth.

Dimensions: Varies

Tips and Pitfalls: Insert with the narrower side of the "V" shape first (ie, aimed toward the posterior molars).

Weitlaner Self-Retaining Retractor

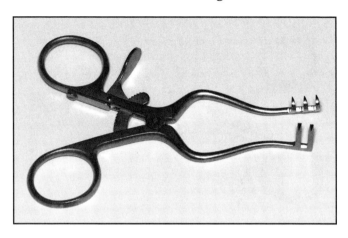

Aliases and Nicknames: Weity (pronounced "wheaty"), self-retainer, Weitlander (a *misnomer* that should not be used as there is no "d" in the true name of the instrument)

Uses: Holding incisions open in a hands-free manner.

Description: Ratcheting retractor with distal tines containing sharp forklike extensions (teeth). Other than tines, this instrument is flat.

Dimensions: 14 cm long

Tips and Pitfalls: Open the retractor so that the handles are facing away from the field and the surgeon (and thus out of the way).

Articulating Weitlaner Self-Retaining Retractor

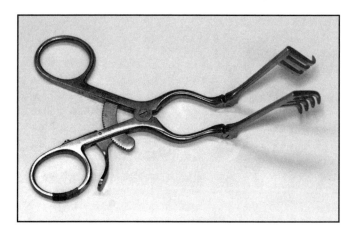

Aliases and Nicknames: See Weitlaner retractor above

Uses: Holding incisions open in a hands-free manner. Unlike the regular Weitlaner, the hinge in the articulating Weitlaner allows the axis of the handle to be adjusted so that the handles are more out of the way of the surgical field.

Description: Ratcheting retractor with distal tines designed to hold incisions open. The axis of the tines is fixed, but there is a hinge in the middle of the instrument so that the handles can be bent in different directions.

Dimensions: 14 cm long

Double-Pronged Hook

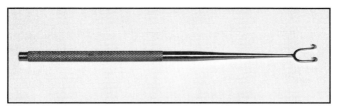

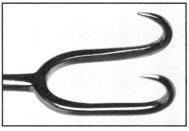

Aliases and Nicknames: Double-prong skin hook

Uses: Retracting skin and other delicate tissues. Can often be used while harvesting full-thickness skin grafts: pull the skin back with this instrument and leave your finger underneath the epidermal side of the skin so that you can always feel the thickness while harvesting.

Description: Narrow handle, tip contains two fine, sharp hooks.

Dimensions: 16 cm long

Tips and Pitfalls: To avoid injury, remember that this is a sharp retractor.

Double-Pronged Hook, Fine

See p. 252.

Single-Pronged Hook

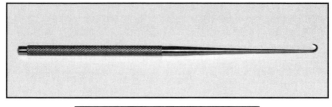

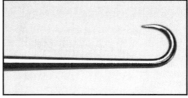

Aliases and Nicknames: Single prong, small hook

Uses: Retracting skin and other delicate tissues.

Description: Narrow handle, tapers to a sharp hook at the tip.

Dimensions: 16 cm long

Tips and Pitfalls: To avoid injury, remember that this is a sharp retractor.

General and Miscellaneous Instruments

Scalpel Handle #3

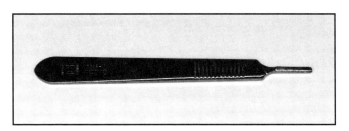

Aliases and Nicknames: Knife, often requested according to the blade attached to the handle (eg, 15 blade, 15)

Uses: Most commonly used scalpel handle, accommodates the most commonly used blades (#10, #11, #12, #15).

Description: Long thin handle with tip that fits snugly into the groove of a disposable scalpel blade

Dimensions: 13 cm long without the blade

Tips and Pitfalls: Avoid injury by applying/removing blades with a clamp (usually scrub personnel will do this). Always use good communication when passing sharps around the field.

Scalpel Handle #7

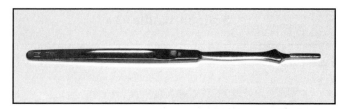

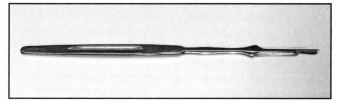

Aliases and Nicknames: Knife, often requested by the blade attached to the handle (eg, 15 blade, 15)

Uses: An alternative to the #3 scalpel handle. Easier to hold like a pencil for more precise cuts or when extended reach is needed. Also accommodates the most commonly used blades (#10, #11, #12, #15).

Description: Long thin/narrow handle with tip that fits snugly into the groove of a disposable scalpel blade (first image). A #7 handle assembled with a #15 blade is also pictured above (second image).

Dimensions: 17 cm long without the blade

Tips and Pitfalls: Avoid injury by applying/removing blades with a clamp (usually the scrub personnel will do this). Always use good communication when passing sharps around the field.

Scalpel Blades #10, #11, #15

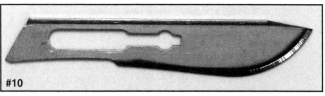

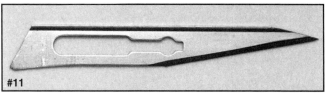

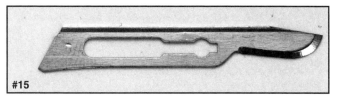

Aliases and Nicknames: Blade, knife. The assembled scalpel (handle and blade) is usually requested by the blade number, eg, 15 blade.

Uses: The #10 blade is used for making very long, straight incisions. The #11 blade is used for making very short stabbing incisions, most commonly for incision and drainage (I&D) of an abscess. It may also be used for removing sutures. The #15 blade is the most commonly used in otolaryngology.

Description: The #10 and #15 cutting surfaces have a similar shape, with the latter being smaller. Both contain a large "belly" and rounding near the tip. The #11 is shaped like a very acute triangle and comes to an extremely fine point.

Tips and Pitfalls: The bellies of the #10 and #15 blades are used for creating the incision. The "point" at the distal-most tip is less commonly used. The #11 blade, in contrast, is used for creating stabbing incisions. The blade is steeply angled to the skin, near perpendicular, and in a controlled stabbing motion is inserted into an abscess cavity. Always use good communication when passing sharps around the field.

Needle Driver

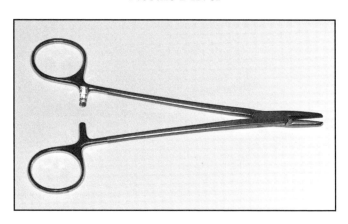

Aliases and Nicknames: Needle holder

Uses: Gripping firmly at a specific part of a suture needle, driving needles through tissue, instrument tying.

Description: Ratcheting clamp mechanism, tips designed to firmly grip suture needles.

Dimensions: Length and caliber vary widely according to the size and type of suture to be used.

Tips and Pitfalls: Be sure that the instrument is clamped tightly enough to hold the needle in place; otherwise, the needle may slip while you are trying to suture. Always use good communication when passing sharps around the field.

Note: For fine or specialized needle drivers, see pp. 292–296.

Vascular Clip Applier

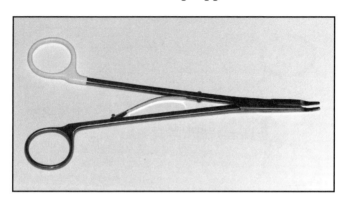

Aliases and Nicknames: Clip, large clip, small clip

Uses: Application of vascular clips to blood vessels.

Description: Ring-handled instrument with small, thin tines designed to hold an open metal clip. Clips of different sizes are available with corresponding clip appliers, which are often color coded for ease of identification.

Dimensions: ~20 cm long (varies)

Tips and Pitfalls: A metal clip is inserted between the tines by scrub personnel. Next, the clip/tines are placed around the vessel or other tissue to be clipped, and then the handles of the instrument are squeezed firmly to apply the clip. Do not squeeze handles at all before ready to apply the clip or it may fall off prematurely. Just before squeezing the handles, be sure that the clip is still in place on the instrument.

Wire Cutters

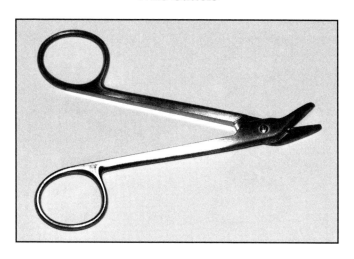

Uses: Cutting wires that are used for orthognathic and reconstructive surgery.

Description: Scissorlike design with heavy, serrated blades designed for cutting wire.

Dimensions: 13 cm long (varies)

Tips and Pitfalls: Cutting thicker-caliber material is easier near the hinge than the tip.

Towel Clamp, Penetrating

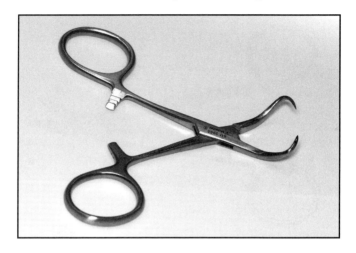

Aliases and Nicknames: Towel clamp, Backhaus towel forceps

Uses: Holding towels, drapes, and other objects in place on the sterile field.

Description: Ratcheting clamp with curved, sharp (penetrating) tips.

Dimensions: ~13 cm long

Tips and Pitfalls: Avoid pinching the patient's face/skin when clamping these on the towels. Avoid using near the eyes.

Towel Clamp, Nonpenetrating

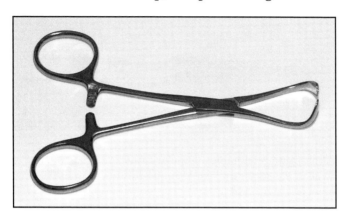

Aliases and Nicknames: Towel clamp

Uses: Same as penetrating towel clamp.

Description: Ratcheting clamps with blunt (nonpenetrating), flared tips with grasping teeth.

Dimensions: ~13 cm long

Tips and Pitfalls: Avoid pinching the patient's face/skin when clamping these on the towels.

Bipolar Cautery Forceps

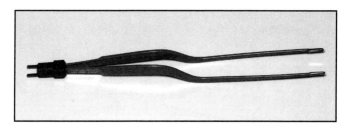

Aliases and Nicknames: Bipolar cautery, bipolar, often will refer to the specific type of bipolar forceps such as bayonet bipolar or Adson bipolar

Uses: Cautery in small, delicate areas or where desirable to avoid using monopolar cautery and spread of current (such as near nerves, other vital structures, or a cochlear implant). May be used just prior to dividing tissue with scissors.

Description: Shaped like various types of traditional forceps (eg, bayonet forceps, as pictured above), with a plug for the cable at the handle apex and cauterizing tips on the other end. Insulated (often in blue coloration) except for the tips.

Dimensions: Varies; bayonet bipolar is 19 cm long, Adson bipolar is 11 cm long

Tips and Pitfalls: Hold the tips of the forceps slightly apart while cauterizing, which allows the current to arc between the tips. Cautery is usually activated with a foot pedal.

Bovie Electrocautery

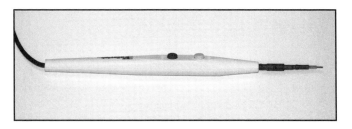

Aliases and Nicknames: Bovie, cautery, monopolar cautery

Uses: Dividing tissue while cauterizing, allowing better hemostasis than a scalpel. Cautery of small vessels to stop bleeding.

Description: Shaped like a pencil with a cable at the handle end and cauterizing tips on the other end. Insulated except for the tip. Tip is interchangeable and numerous styles are available. Contains "cut" and "coag" (coagulate) modes, with the latter mode allowing better hemostasis at the expense of more thermal injury. The cut and coag modes may be activated with a finger switch (as pictured above) or foot petal.

Dimensions: Varies

Tips and Pitfalls: Never bury the tip of the instrument when activated. Hold the tip slightly away from tissue when cauterizing for pinpoint bleeding. This creates a current arc, allowing for better hemostasis.

Suction Bovie Electrocautery

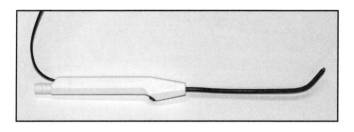

Aliases and Nicknames: Suction Bovie

Uses: Commonly used for adenoidectomy, hemostasis after tonsillectomy, and sinonasal surgery. Useful for cautery during active bleeding when the field is not large enough to accommodate a standard suction at the same time as a standard Bovie. During adenoidectomy, used for simultaneous cautery and suction of adenoid fragments.

Description: Similar to standard Bovie electrocautery but with a hollow lumen hooked up to a suction line. The tip is thus cylindrical and also not interchangeable. Occluding the finger hole in the handle increases suction power. The neck is malleable, allowing one to work around corners (eg, accessing the nasopharynx transorally). Cautery may be activated by a finger button (as pictured above) or a foot pedal.

Dimensions: Varies

Tips and Pitfalls: Hold the tip at an angle slightly away from tissue when cauterizing for pinpoint bleeding. This creates a current arc, allowing for better hemostasis.

Yankauer Suction

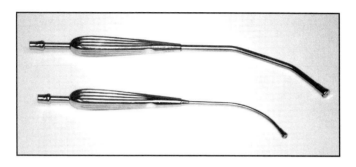

Aliases and Nicknames: Yankauer, Yankauer suction tube, smaller size often called baby Yankhauer or pediatric Yankhauer

Uses: Suctioning in larger fields.

Description: Large, hollow, handled instrument with a flared tip and a bent neck. The tip contains multiple holes. Suction tubing connects at the handle end. There is no finger hole on the handle to modulate the suction power. May be made of surgical steel (as pictured above) or plastic.

Dimensions: Varies

Tips and Pitfalls: When assisting, always suction where the surgeon is working. Do not get distracted by suctioning pools of blood off the field. When suctioning an oozing vessel just prior to cautery, it is helpful to slowly come away allowing the bleeding site to be identified. The Bovie can then quickly be applied to this site before blood reaccumulates.

Frazier Suction, Baron Suction

See pp. 71–72.

McCabe Facial Nerve Dissector

See p. 297.

Instruments for Robotic Surgery

Feyh-Kastenbauer Laryngopharyngoscope
(With Attachments)

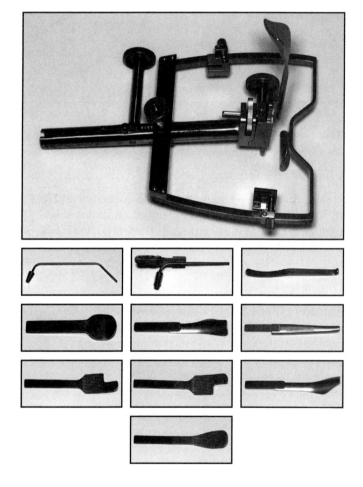

Aliases and Nicknames: FK retractor

Uses: Used in the oral cavity for transoral robotic surgery (TORS) to retract the cheeks and tongue. It is designed to retract tissue in three dimensions. Also can be used when repairing a Zenker's diverticulum.

Description: Large retractor with a self-retaining, ratcheting mechanism and a variety of suction/smoke evacuation, retraction, and laryngopharyngoscope attachments that can be attached to the two sides or to the center bar.

Dimensions: This is the largest of oral retractors/mouth gags. The attachments vary in size/length.

Da Vinci Robot EndoWrist Instruments

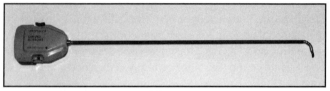

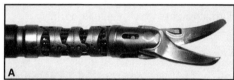

A

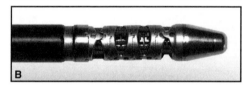

B

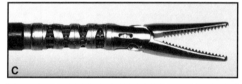

C

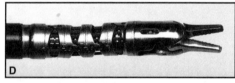

D

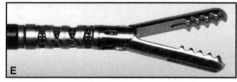

E

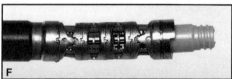

F

Uses: These are connected to the da Vinci system for use in transoral robotic surgery (TORS) or robotic thyroid surgery.

Description: The controls that interface with the machine are housed in the proximal plastic box (on left in first image), which contains 4 wheels connected to cables that extend down the shaft to the instrument tip. Several instruments are commonly used:

A: Curved Scissors

B: 5 French Introducer (to introduce laser)

C: Maryland Dissector (for grasping/dissecting)

D: Needle Driver

E: Schertel Grasper (for grasping/dissecting)

F: Monopolar Cautery (a disposable spatula tip, which
is not pictured, connects to the white plastic connector
shown above)

Dimensions: These instruments are 5-mm EndoWrist instruments; alternative 8-mm instruments are also available.

Kuppersmith Robotic Thyroidectomy Retractor Set

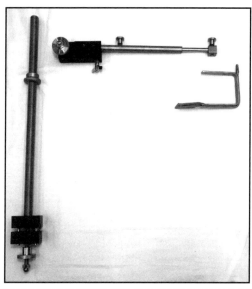

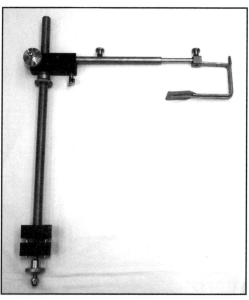

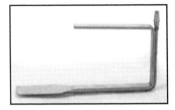 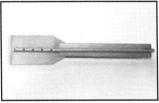

Close-up photos courtesy of Marina Medical

Uses: Retraction of the chest wall during transaxillary robotic-assisted thyroidectomy.

Description: Consists of a table post and clamp for suspension from the table, with a horizontal extension bar and coupler (disassembled, first image; assembled, second image). The coupler then holds the Kuppersmith retractor (side view, third image; inferior view, fourth image; other sizes are also available), which is then suspended while retracting the axillary/chest wall tissue superiorly. Each interchangeable retractor has a suction port for hands-free smoke evacuation.

Dimensions: Table post and clamp measure 22 cm, and the height can be adjusted up to 10 cm. Horizontal extension bar measures 21.5 cm, and can be adjusted to various heights along the table post. The Kuppersmith retractor measures 50 to 70 mm (varies).

CHAPTER

Otologic and Neurotologic Surgery

Justin S. Golub, Jay T. Rubinstein, and Kathleen C. Y. Sie

CONTENTS

Periosteal Elevators
Lempert Elevator
Joseph Elevator
Freer Elevator
Gimmick Elevator
Duckbill Elevator (Large and Small)

Forceps and Scissors
Alligator Forceps
Bellucci Scissors (Curved and Straight; Large and Small)
House-Dieter Malleus Nipper
Large Ear Cup Forceps (Straight, Left, Right)
Mini Ear Cup Forceps (Straight, Left, Right)
Micro Ear Cup Forceps (Straight, Left, Right, Up)
Sheehy Ossicle Holding Clamp
Jeweler's Forceps
Electrode Claw
Cup Bayonet Forceps

Curettes
Mastoid Curette
House Double-Ended Curette
Angled Microcurette
Cerumen Curette
Cerumen Loop
Rongeur

Tissue Presses and Carving Blocks
Fascia Press
Paparella Tissue Press
Carving Block

Microsurgical Knives, Picks, and Rasps
Rosen Needle
Straight Pick
Angled Straight Pick
Incudostapedial Joint Knife

Round Knife (Large, Small)
Lancet Knife
Oval Window Raspatory (Large, Small)
Tabb Myringoplasty Knife (25°/45°)
Tabb Myringoplasty Knife (90°/115–120°)
McCabe Flap Knife Dissector
Whirlybird Knife (Right and Left)
Sickle Knife
Myringotomy Knife
Vertical Roller Knife
Horizontal Roller Knife
Measuring Rod
Strut Caliper and Measuring Gauge
Fisch Raspatory (Left and Right)

Telescopes and Mirrors
Middle Ear Telescope
Large Buckingham Mirror
Small Buckingham Mirror

Drills
Otologic Drill
Microdrill

Miscellaneous Instruments
NIM (Nerve Integrity Monitor) Incrementing
Probe, Prass Tip

Specula and Retractors

Lempert Speculum

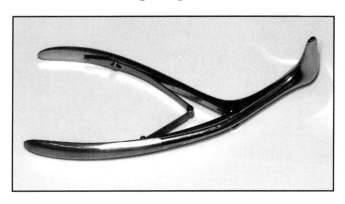

Aliases and Nicknames: Lempert

Uses: Examining the external auditory canal and tympanic membrane.

Description: Similar to a nasal speculum, but with a curved neck and flatter blades.

Dimensions: 20 cm long

Aural Speculum

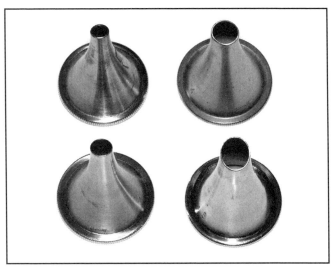

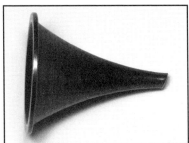

Aliases and Nicknames: Ear speculum

Uses: Examining the external auditory canal and tympanic membrane.

Description: Tip is often beveled. Many sizes and style variations are available.

Dimensions: Varies

Tips and Pitfalls: When the tip is beveled, the longer part (top of tip in second image) should be directed anteriorly.

Use the largest size possible for maximal visualization. May then upsize progressively (ie, dilating) as allowed. When dictating an operative report, often need to spell out "aural" or will be transcribed as "oral." Speculum holders exist to aid when using for transcanal approaches.

Self-Retaining Retractor

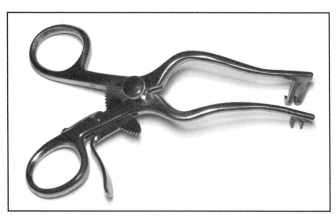

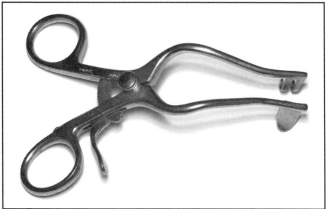

Aliases and Nicknames: Numerous subtypes including Wullstein, Bellucci-Wullstein, Weitlaner, Paparella-Weitlaner, Schucknect-Weitlaner, House, Perkins

Uses: Retraction of soft tissue for exposure of the mastoid cortex.

Description: Unlike a standard Weitlaner self-retaining retractor (see p. 37), many retractors used for otologic surgery feature an angled neck, which permits easier placement on the curved lateral cranium. Various teeth styles are available, including sharp and dull with configurations including 3×3 prongs, 3×1, 2×2, 2×1, etc. A *Bellucci-Wullstein retractor* has 2 prongs × 1 dull plate (second image above). A *Perkins retractor* has 3 prongs × 1 L-shaped plate (not pictured). A *Wullstein retractor* has 3×3 sharp prongs (not pictured).

Dimensions: Size varies widely.

Tips and Pitfalls: Engage the prongs in the periosteal flaps before opening them. For mastoid surgery, often use two retractors at right angles to one another for improved exposure. Positioning the handles away from the surgeon (eg, one pair anteriorly and one pair superiorly) places them out of the way. Some surgeons will begin with a standard straight Weitlaner retractor and then change to an angled self-retaining retractor later. Retractors with plates instead of prongs are designed to avoid trauma to soft tissue flaps.

Janetta Retractor

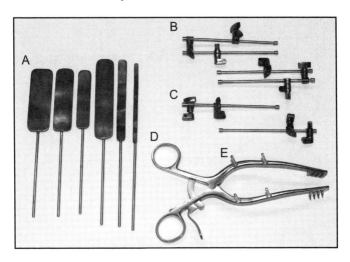

Uses: Retraction of the cerebellar dura during lateral skull base procedures, such as translabyrinthine approach to the cerebellopontine angle.

Description: Contains a self-retaining retractor (**D**) with four pins (**E**) on the arms. Double (**B**) or single (**C**) bars sit on the pins and attach to flat retractor blades (**A**) that retract the brain. The retractor blades are malleable.

House-Urban Middle Fossa Retractor

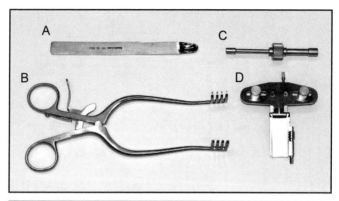

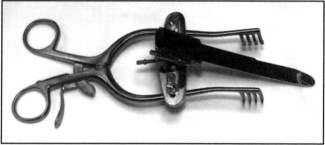

Aliases and Nicknames: Middle fossa retractor, temporal lobe retractor

Uses: Retraction of the temporal lobe dura during middle cranial fossa approaches.

Description: Contains a self-retaining retractor (**B**) onto which a hinged adapter (**D**) sits. A blade (**A**) slides into the hinged adapter and superomedially displaces the temporal lobe. The hinged adapter contains several screws and pins that allow adjustment of the exposure. Adjustments are made with the aid of a specialized wrench (**C**). The assembled retractor appears in the second image.

Suction and Irrigation

Frazier Suction, Baron Suction

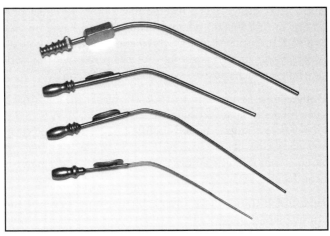

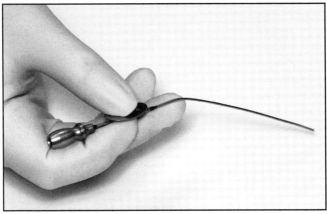

Aliases and Nicknames: Frazier, Frazier suction tube, Frazier tip suction, Frazier tip, Baron, Baron suction tube. Often referred to by the size in French (ie, number 7 suction, 7 Frazier).

Uses: Suctioning in small areas (eg, ear canal, middle ear, mastoid, nose), or in delicate head and neck procedures. Also used for placement of grafts, Gelfoam, or other materials.

Description: Small thin tubular shaft with a bend and a proximal thumb plate with a hole. Ends proximally with an olive-shaped or grooved prominence that connects to the plastic/rubber suction line. Tip has one hole at the distal end. *Frazier* design has a rectangular thumb plate (suction on top in first image) whereas *Baron* design has a thinner ovular thumb plate (bottom three suctions in first image). A *Brackmann* suction is similar but has a rounded tip with side holes, which causes less trauma (not pictured).

Dimensions: Sizing unit is *French*. The most commonly used sizes (diameters) are 8 (more for nasal surgery), 7, 5, and 3 French (shown top to bottom in first image). (In French system, larger numbers indicate larger diameters whereas in gauge system, larger numbers indicate smaller diameters.) Lengths vary.

Tips and Pitfalls: Place thumb on the holed side of the thumb plate and index finger on the opposite side. The third finger may be used to stabilize the shaft at the bend (see second image). When suctioning delicate areas, use without thumb over the thumb plate hole, which decreases the suction power. By alternately sealing and unsealing the thumb plate hole, it is possible to pick up and then let go of small material such as Gelfoam. Typically, this is accomplished with a second instrument to place various materials or grafts into the middle ear. For delicate work, may attach a rubber suction line, which has more flexibility than a plastic suction line.

Microsuction

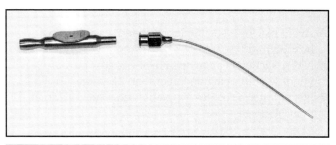

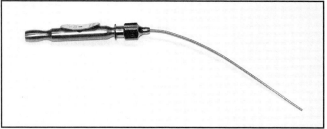

Aliases and Nicknames: Often referred to by the size in gauge (eg, 20 gauge suction, 20 suction)

Uses: Suctioning in very small areas.

Description: Similar to Baron suction, except smaller diameter. The thumb plate is part of a separate component called the *House cutoff adapter* (component on left in first image). The suction tube component is called a *Rosen suction tube* (component on the right in first image). The House cutoff adapter is universal; however, the Rosen suction tubes are available in many sizes.

Dimensions: Unlike Frazier and Baron suctions, sizing unit is *gauge*. Common sizes (diameters) are 20, 22, and 24 gauge. (In French system, larger numbers indicate larger diameters. In gauge system, larger numbers indicate smaller diameters.) The Rosen suction tube pictured is 11 cm long.

Tips and Pitfalls: A 20 gauge suction is slightly smaller than a 3 French suction. When suctioning near the stapedial footplate, do not put your finger over the thumb hole. General rules for suction size limits:

- Avoid placing a suction larger than 20 gauge into a hearing middle ear.
- Never suction near an open oval window or round window with a suction larger than 24 gauge.
- Never touch a cochlear implant with a suction larger than 24 gauge.

Microirrigation

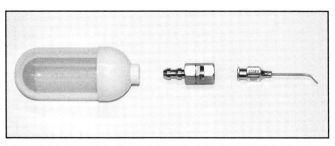

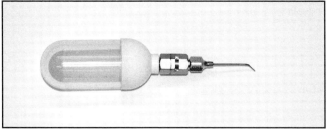

Aliases and Nicknames: Irrigation

Uses: Irrigating in very small areas.

Description: Consists of a small, compressible irrigation bottle (component on left in first image), an adapter (component in middle), and a short irrigation tube (component on right).

Tips and Pitfalls: Lightly squeezing the irrigation bottle will gently release irrigant. The adapter will also accommodate irrigation through a Rosen suction tube (see p. 73).

House Suction Irrigator

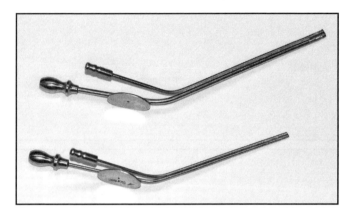

Aliases and Nicknames: Suction irrigator

Uses: Irrigating and suctioning the surgical field simultaneously with a single instrument. (Alternatively, irrigation may be integrated into the drill; see Otologic Drill on pp. 120–121). Commonly used while drilling.

Description: Consists of a Baron-type suction (see pp. 71–72) with an additional irrigation port. The shafts of the suction and irrigation components are fused. The proximal end of the suction component connects to a suction line and the proximal end of the irrigation component connects to an irrigation line. Pictured above are sizes 8 French (top) and 5 French (bottom).

Dimensions: Sizing unit is *French*. Size varies and numerous diameters are available.

Tips and Pitfalls: Speed of irrigation is controlled by adjusting clamping over the irrigation line tubing (typically by the scrub technician/nurse). For the surgeon to directly control the irrigation speed, consider the Essar suction irrigator (see next entry).

Essar Suction Irrigator

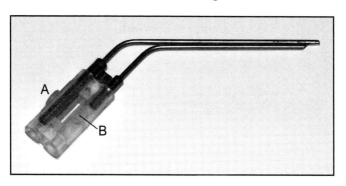

Aliases and Nicknames: Suction irrigator

Uses: Same as House suction irrigator.

Description: Handle includes a rubber sheath. The top portion of the sheath (A) contains a suction thumb hole. The side button (B) allows control of the irrigation flow rate.

Dimensions: Sizing unit is *French*. Size varies and numerous diameters available from 4-19 French.

Tips and Pitfalls: Unlike the simpler House suction irrigator, this device allows the surgeon to control the speed of the irrigation directly. Similar to the House suction irrigator, occluding the thumb hole (A) increases the suction power. Squeezing the side irrigation button (B), which can be done with the third and fourth fingers, allows the surgeon to increase the flow of irrigation.

Periosteal Elevators

Lempert Elevator

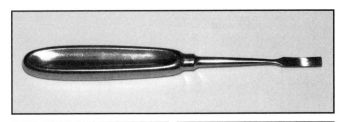

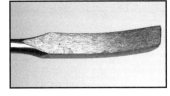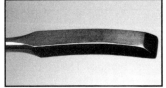

Aliases and Nicknames: Lempert

Uses: Elevating periosteum from bone. Commonly used to elevate periosteum from the mastoid cortex and temporal squamosa before mastoidectomy.

Description: Broad handle. The tip has a slight concavity. The distal tip is squared and tapers to a fine edge.

Dimensions: 18 cm long

Tips and Pitfalls: It is helpful to hold this instrument with both hands and pivot around your nondominant hand. As such, the instrument is often held nearly perpendicular to the bone. Do not use when elevating soft tissue in more delicate areas, such as the external auditory canal. A similar instrument, which is often used for dissecting dura off the floor of the middle cranial fossa, is the *Adson periosteal elevator* (nicknamed *the joker*). The Lempert elevator may also be used for this purpose.

Joseph Elevator

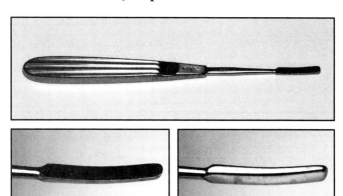

Aliases and Nicknames: Joseph

Uses: Elevating soft tissue from bone and cartilage in more delicate regions, such as the external auditory canal, or where more precision is needed than with the Lempert.

Description: Smaller than the Lempert elevator. The tip has a slight concavity. The tip is also smaller than the Lempert elevator's, and is rounded, rather than squared.

Dimensions: 17 cm long

Tips and Pitfalls: Not ideal for elevating tissue on the mastoid cortex because of smaller size. Often used for elevating tissue from the bony external auditory meatus. Unlike the Lempert, this periosteal elevator is used in a more typical pushing fashion. As such, the instrument is held at an acute angle to the bone.

Freer Elevator

See p. 284.

Gimmick Elevator

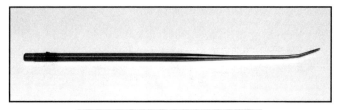

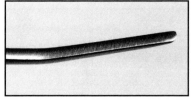

Aliases and Nicknames: Annulus elevator, Gimmick

Uses: Raising a tympanomeatal flap, particularly when elevating the annulus.

Description: Thin octagonal handle. Tip is angled 15°. One surface of the tip is flat and the other is rounded. Tip narrows to a broad point to allow elevation off bone.

Dimensions: 17 cm long

Tips and Pitfalls: After elevating the annulus may switch to a smaller elevator, such as the duckbill elevator.

Duckbill Elevator (Large and Small)

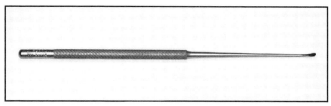

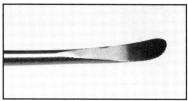

Aliases and Nicknames: Large (or small) duckbill

Uses: Raising flaps in more delicate regions.

Description: Tip is rounded, slightly concave, and broadly narrows at distal end. Both large and small tip sizes are available.

Dimensions: 16 cm long

Tips and Pitfalls: May be used in the external auditory canal and middle ear.

Forceps and Scissors

Alligator Forceps

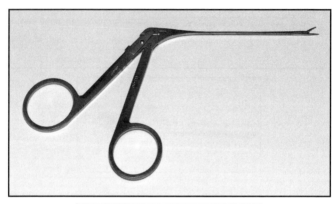

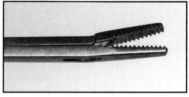

Aliases and Nicknames: Alligator

Uses: Grasping delicate soft tissue and other small materials or objects.

Description: Pistol-grip handle with finely serrated grasping tip.

Dimensions: 14 cm long

Tips and Pitfalls: Before grasping critical structures (such as components of a cochlear implant), verify that the tips are those of alligator forceps and not Bellucci scissors. The instruments look similar under nonmicroscopic vision and may be confused (ie, the scrub personnel might accidentally hand the surgeon the wrong instrument, leading to inadvertent cutting of a structure).

Bellucci Scissors
(Curved and Straight; Large and Small)

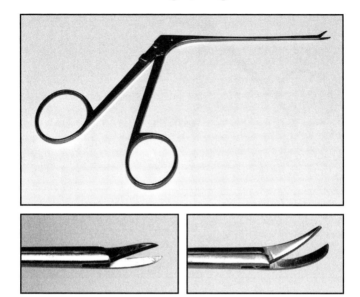

Aliases and Nicknames: (Large/small, left curved/right curved/straight) Bellucci scissors; large Bellucci also called regular Bellucci, small Bellucci also called micro Bellucci

Uses: For cutting small soft tissue, for example the stapedial tendon.

Description: Pistol-grip handle with small, sharp, nonserrated cutting edge. Tips may be straight (second image), curved right (third image), or curved left. Tips also come in smaller and larger sizes.

Dimensions: 14 cm long

Tips and Pitfalls: May rarely be confused with alligator forceps (see previous entry).

House-Dieter Malleus Nipper

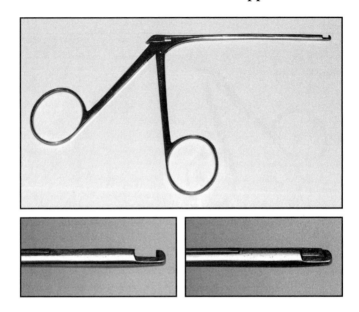

Aliases and Nicknames: Malleus nipper

Uses: Cutting the malleus neck to allow removal of the malleus head.

Description: Pistol-grip handle with a sliding action tip. Second image depicts tip open, third image depicts tip closed.

Dimensions: 14 cm long

Large Ear Cup Forceps (Straight, Left, Right)

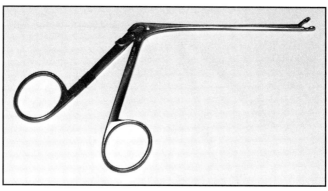

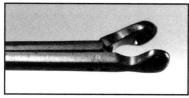

Aliases and Nicknames: Large cup (straight, left, right).

Uses: Grasping tissue or objects.

Description: Pistol-grip handle with large cupped tips. Tips may be straight, angled left, or angled right.

Dimensions: 14 cm long

Mini Ear Cup Forceps (Straight, Left, Right)

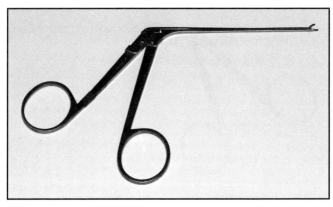

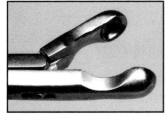 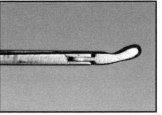

Aliases and Nicknames: Small cup, mini cup straight (or left, or right, as applicable)

Uses: Grasping smaller and more delicate tissue and objects.

Description: Pistol-grip handle with tips straight, to the left (third image above from superior view), or to the right.

Dimensions: 14 cm long

Micro Ear Cup Forceps (Straight, Left, Right, Up)

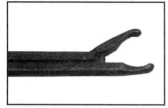 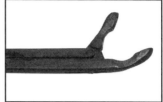

Aliases and Nicknames: Micro cup (straight, left, right, up)

Uses: Grasping extremely small or delicate tissue and objects.

Description: Pistol-grip handle with cups smaller than in the mini cupped forceps. May be traditional angle (first image) or angled up (second image). Left and right may also be available.

Sheehy Ossicle Holding Clamp

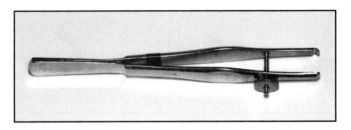

Aliases and Nicknames: Ossicle holding clamp, incus clamp

Uses: Holding the incus while shaping it for incus interposition graft.

Description: Basic forceps design with medial concavity on both tips. Contains a thumbscrew near the distal end for tightening.

Dimensions: 12 cm long

Tips and Pitfalls: May also be used as a clamp on the irrigation line to control the rate of irrigation.

Jeweler's Forceps

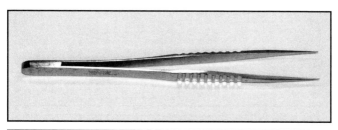

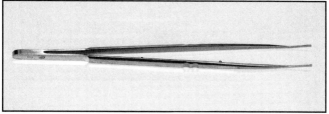

Aliases and Nicknames: Jeweler's. The forceps in the second image may be called AOS (advance off-stylet) forceps, modified jeweler's forceps, or implant forceps.

Uses: Grasping delicate structures, such as the electrode array of a cochlear implant.

Description: Forceps with fine tips. The first image depicts standard jeweler's forceps with tips coming to a point. The second image depicts a modified jeweler's forceps (manufactured by Cochlear) with a curved distal end and subtly cupped tips that do not come to a point. The modified tips are designed to gently cup the cochlear implant electrode array while minimizing rotation.

Dimensions: Varies; forceps in first image are 12 cm long, forceps in second image are 15 cm long.

Electrode Claw

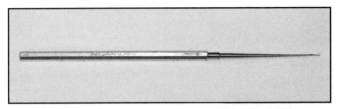

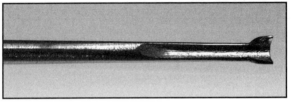

Aliases and Nicknames: Claw, Contour electrode claw

Uses: Inserting cochlear implant electrode array into the cochlea or positioning a ground electrode.

Description: Straight handle and shaft. Tip contains a claw-like groove for gently advancing the electrode array into the cochlea.

Cup Bayonet Forceps

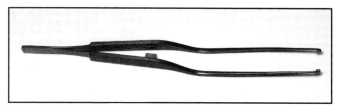

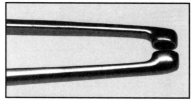

Aliases and Nicknames: Cup bayonet

Uses: Removal of skull base tumors.

Description: Similar to a standard bayonet forceps, except with cupped tips. The above model is made out of light-weight titanium.

Dimensions: ~20 cm long

Curettes

Mastoid Curette

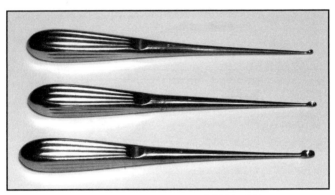

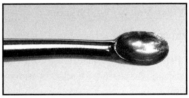

Aliases and Nicknames: Curette

Uses: Removal of bone including in the mastoid and the spine of Henle.

Description: Large, long handle with a small tip to allow the surgeon to use the instrument in small spaces with precision but adequate force.

Dimensions: 20–21 cm long. Various size tips (as pictured above).

Tips and Pitfalls: Use rotary motion to remove bone (think of twisting the wrist).

House Double-Ended Curette

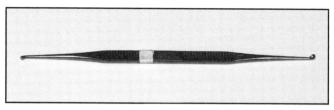

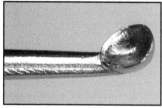
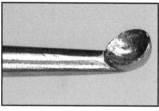

Aliases and Nicknames: Curettes with different tip configurations are lettered. Usually referred to by the letter, with the most common being the *K curette*.

Uses: Removal of bone in smaller regions (eg, taking down the scutum).

Description: Ridged shaft that acts as handle, ends contain a larger (second image) and smaller (third image) cup-shaped curette. Available in multiple tip sizes. The K curette is pictured above.

Dimensions: 15 cm long

Angled Microcurette

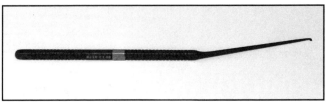

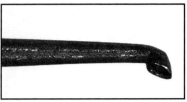

Uses: Removal of bone in the middle ear.

Description: More delicate than a House double-ended curette, angled at distal handle.

Dimensions: 15 cm long

Cerumen Curette

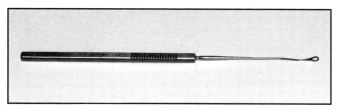

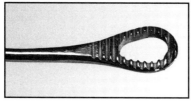

Aliases and Nicknames: Curette

Uses: Removal of cerumen from the external auditory canal.

Description: Long, thin handle with ridged circular tip. The neck is malleable.

Dimensions: 16 cm long, tip size varies

Tips and Pitfalls: Use gently; like the cerumen loop (see next entry), can easily damage the delicate skin of the bony external auditory canal.

Cerumen Loop

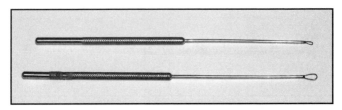

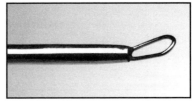

Aliases and Nicknames: Ear loop

Uses: Removal of cerumen from the external auditory canal.

Description: Long, thin handle with gently curved malleable wire loop at tip.

Dimensions: ~16 cm long, tip size varies

Tips and Pitfalls: Use gently; like the cerumen curette (see previous entry), this instrument can still easily damage the delicate skin of the external auditory canal.

Rongeur

See pp. 271–272.

Tissue Presses and Carving Blocks

Fascia Press

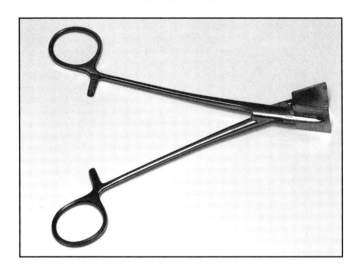

Aliases and Nicknames: Press

Uses: Compressing (temporalis) fascia for use in tympanic membrane grafting. Also used for compressing Gelfoam or perichondrium.

Description: Similar to a hemostat, except the distal end has two plates for compressing fascia. The proximal end has a ratcheted locking mechanism.

Dimensions: 19 cm long

Paparella Tissue Press

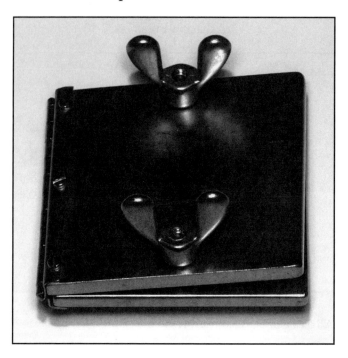

Aliases and Nicknames: Fascia press, press

Uses: Compressing (temporalis) fascia for use in tympanic membrane grafting. Also used for compressing Gelfoam or perichondrium.

Description: Consists of two heavy metal plates bound by a hinge. Two metal hand screws permit tightening of the plates to compress their contents.

Dimensions: 7 × 7 cm

Carving Block

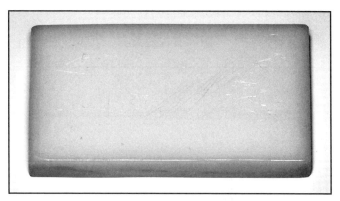

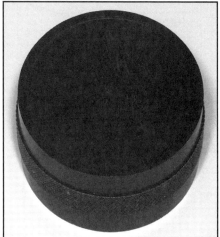

Aliases and Nicknames: Cutting block

Uses: Carving fascia or cartilage grafts (eg, for tympanic membrane reconstruction).

Description: Several styles are available including rectangular (first image) and a cylindrical Teflon block with a knurled waist (second image).

Dimensions: Varies

Microsurgical Knives, Picks, and Rasps

Rosen Needle

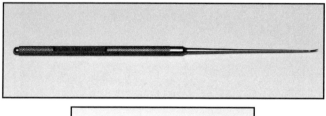

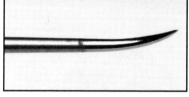

Aliases and Nicknames: Rosen pick, Rosen

Uses: Palpating, repositioning of objects. Commonly used to precisely position a tympanostomy tube into the myringotomy after using the alligator forceps. May also be used to palpate the ossicular chain for mobility.

Description: Straight handle and shaft. Distal tip is curved and comes to a point.

Dimensions: 17 cm long

Straight Pick

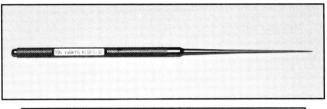

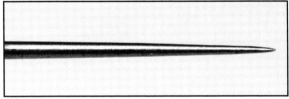

Uses: Middle ear dissection.

Description: Straight handle and shaft. Tip is straight and comes to a point.

Dimensions: 17 cm long

Angled Straight Pick

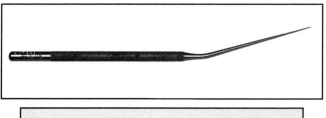

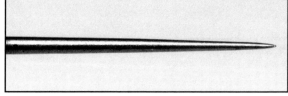

Aliases and Nicknames: Angled straight

Uses: Middle ear dissection.

Description: Similar to the straight pick but with an obtuse angle at the distal handle.

Dimensions: 17 cm long

Tips and Pitfalls: Angled instruments offset the tip from the handle, which can reduce the surgeon's fingers from getting into the field of view.

Incudostapedial Joint Knife

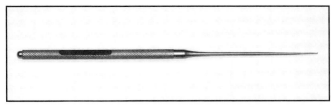

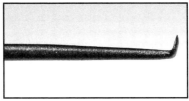

Aliases and Nicknames: IS joint knife

Uses: Disarticulating the incus from the stapes.

Description: Straight instrument with very small distal hook.

Dimensions: 17 cm long

Round Knife (Large, Small)

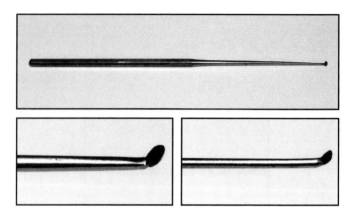

Aliases and Nicknames: (Large or small) weapon, Sheehy knife curette, Sheehy weapon, canal knife

Uses: Numerous purposes, including making incisions in the external auditory canal and elevating a tympanomeatal flap.

Description: Straight handle and shaft with an angled circular blade at the tip. Blades come in large (first and second images) and small (third image) sizes. Distinguished from the lancet knife because blade is circular, whereas lancet is more triangular.

Dimensions: 17 cm long

Lancet Knife

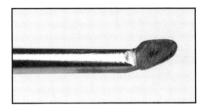

Aliases and Nicknames: #2 knife (Sickle knife is called #1 knife)

Uses: Similar to large round knife.

Description: Straight handle and shaft (similar to round knife). Tip is larger than in the large round knife. The blade is also angled but more triangular shaped.

Dimensions: 17 cm long

Oval Window Raspatory (Large, Small)

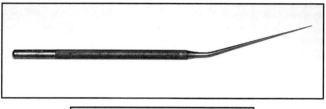

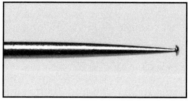

Aliases and Nicknames: Oval window rasp, McGee rasp, Farrior rasp, stapes pick, footplate pick, mushroom pick

Uses: Enlarging a stapedotomy, enlarging a chochleostomy during cochlear implantation.

Description: Obtuse angle at the distal handle. Tip is extremely small and mushroom shaped.

Dimensions: 16 cm long

Tips and Pitfalls: Because of the circular tip can be used to remove bone in any direction.

Tabb Myringoplasty Knife (25°/45°)

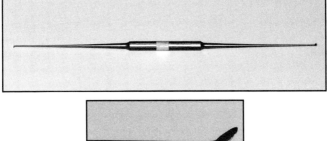

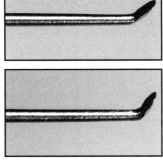

Aliases and Nicknames: Barely bent Tabb knife, barely bent

Uses: Elevation of fine tissue such as a layer off the tympanic membrane or medial canal wall skin in a child.

Description: Central cylindrical handle. Each end contains a bent flat plate with a relatively sharp tip that is slightly ("barely") angulated. One end is less angulated (second image, 25°) than the other (third image, 45°).

Dimensions: 16 cm long

Tabb Myringoplasty Knife (90°/115–120°)

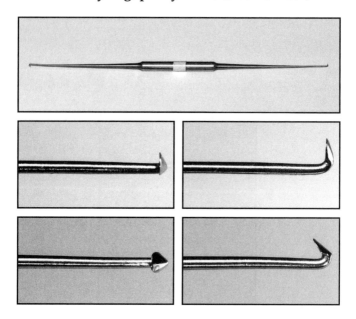

Aliases and Nicknames: Very bent Tabb knife, very bent

Uses: Elevation of fine tissue.

Description: Central cylindrical handle. Each end contains a bent flat plate that is more ("very") angulated compared to the barely bent Tabb knife. One end is at a 90° angle (second image superior view, third image lateral view) and the other end is at a 115° or 120° angle (fourth image superior view, fifth image lateral view).

Dimensions: 16 cm long

McCabe Flap Knife Dissector

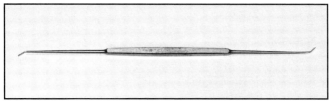

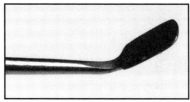

Aliases and Nicknames: McCabe

Uses: Multiple uses. Examples include elevating the tympanic membrane, separating facial nerve from cholesteatoma or vestibular schwannoma, opening the endolymphatic sac.

Description: Contains two tips, each with a small, very thin angled flat plate. The distal-most end of the tip is dull, whereas the sides are sharp. The tip on one side of the instrument is more angulated (45°) than the other (25°).

Dimensions: 18 cm long

Whirlybird Knife (Right and Left)

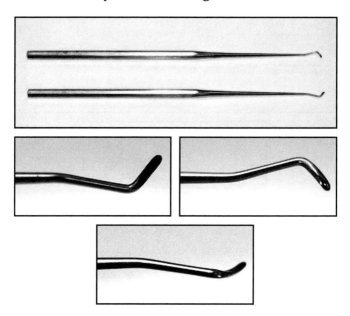

Aliases and Nicknames: Whirlybird

Uses: Elevating tissue, such as out of curved recesses including the epitympanum, facial recess, or sinus tympani.

Description: Tip has multiple bends. Sequence of closeup images above depicts the instrument rotating clockwise.

Dimensions: 16 cm long

Sickle Knife

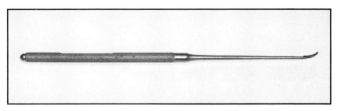

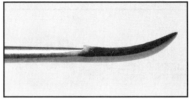

Aliases and Nicknames: #1 knife (Lancet knife is called #2 knife)

Uses: Multiple uses, including cutting the tensor tympani, making inferior part of a tympanomeatal flap, separating the incudostapedial joint, elevating the chorda tympani nerve.

Description: Straight handle, tip is a sickle-shaped blade. Various sized blades are available.

Dimensions: 17 cm long

Myringotomy Knife

See pp. 247–248.

Vertical Roller Knife

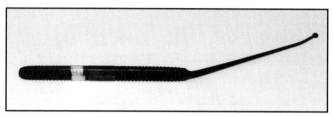

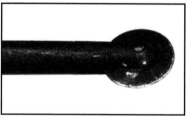

Aliases and Nicknames: Vertical pizza cutter, roller knife with in-line blade

Uses: Making incisions in the external auditory canal.

Description: Ridged handle. Tip contains a circular blade styled like a pizza cutter.

Dimensions: 15 cm long

Tips and Pitfalls: Blade may become dull.

Horizontal Roller Knife

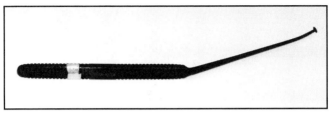

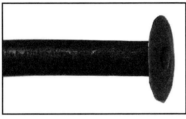

Aliases and Nicknames: Horizontal pizza cutter, roller knife with angled 90° blade

Uses: Making incisions in the external auditory canal.

Description: Similar to vertical roller knife except with transverse blade.

Dimensions: 15 cm long

Tips and Pitfalls: Blade may become dull.

Measuring Rod

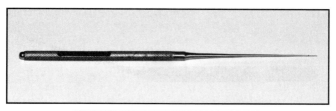

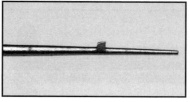

Uses: Measuring the distance between the stapedial foot-plate and the undersurface of the incus. Used during ossiculoplasty and stapedectomy.

Description: Finlike projection near the tip. The distance between the tip and the finlike projection is a specific value, which varies from instrument to instrument. Several sizes and styles are available. Shaft may be malleable.

Dimensions: 17 cm long

Strut Caliper and Measuring Gauge

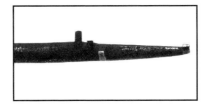

Uses: Similar to measuring rod.

Description: Similar to measuring rod but contains multiple "fins." One common configuration is 4.5, 5.0, and 5.5 mm from each fin to the tip.

Dimensions: 16 cm long

Fisch Raspatory (Left and Right)

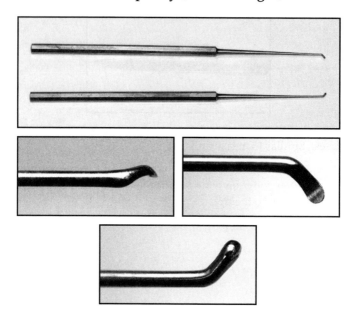

Aliases and Nicknames: Fisch instrument, Fisch left, Fisch right, rasp

Uses: Removing bone off the internal auditory canal or facial nerve.

Description: Straight handle. Tip has multiple bends. Made of strong metal to allow application of relatively large force. Sequence of closeup images above depicts the instrument rotating counterclockwise.

Dimensions: 16 cm long

Tips and Pitfalls: A raspatory is an instrument used for scraping or coarsely filing bone.

Telescopes and Mirrors

Middle Ear Telescope

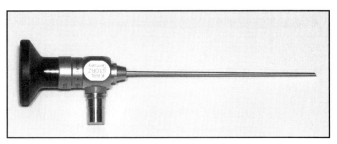

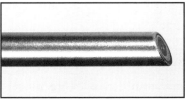

Aliases and Nicknames: Middle ear scope

Uses: For examining regions of the middle ear that are not in direct line of sight, particularly the facial recess, sinus tympani, and epitympanum, to detect residual cholesteatoma.

Description: Rigid Hopkins rod telescope with relatively narrow and short shaft, 30° angled tip.

Dimensions: 15 cm long

Tips and Pitfalls: Some surgeons prefer the middle ear telescope to the Buckingham mirror (see next entry) because of superior optics. Be careful to avoid inadvertent trauma to ossicles when using in the middle ear. For more information about Hopkins rigid telescopes, see p. 127–129.

Large Buckingham Mirror

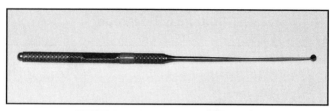

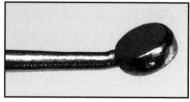

Aliases and Nicknames: Large middle ear mirror

Uses: For examining regions of the middle ear that are not in direct line of sight, particularly the facial recess, sinus tympani, and epitympanum, to detect residual cholesteatoma.

Description: Reflective mirrored surface at tip. Angled at distal neck, straight shaft and handle.

Dimensions: 17 cm long

Tips and Pitfalls: Some surgeons prefer the middle ear telescope (see previous entry) because of superior optics.

Small Buckingham Mirror

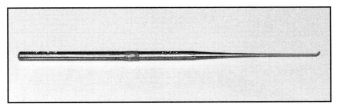

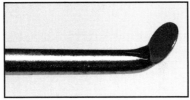

Aliases and Nicknames: Small middle ear mirror

Uses: See large Buckingham mirror (previous entry).

Description: Reflective mirrored surface at tip. Tip is thinner and of smaller diameter than the large Buckingham mirror. Angled at distal neck, straight shaft and handle.

Dimensions: 17 cm long

Tips and Pitfalls: See large Buckingham mirror.

Drills

Otologic Drill

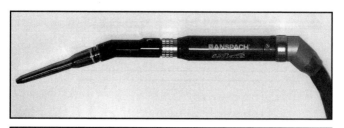

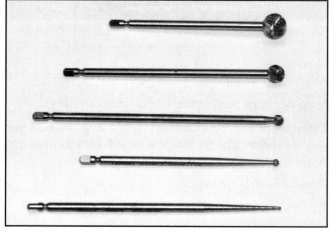

Aliases and Nicknames: Drill, electric (or pneumatic) drill, may be referred to by company name (eg, Anspach drill, as pictured above)

Uses: Drilling through temporal bone, such as during mastoidectomy.

Description: Drills may be electric (as pictured above) or pneumatic. Rotational speed is controlled with a foot pedal. Note that the first image depicts the drill without a bur (bit). In this pictured model, manufactured by Anspach, the base of the drill handle allows free rotation of the electrical tubing. Some models allow irrigation to be attached to the drill itself. Numerous bur sizes and types are available, including cutting (fluted in appearance), rough (or coarse) diamond, and smooth diamond. Sizes indicate the diameter in mm. In the second image, from top to bottom, burs are 7 mm cutting, 5 cutting, 3 cutting, 2 coarse diamond, 1 cutting.

Dimensions: Drill and bur dimensions vary

Tips and Pitfalls: Electric drills tend to be quieter, pneumatic drills tend to be more powerful (more torque). Newer electric models are similar to pneumatic drills in power, however. Cutting burs remove bone faster. Diamond burs are employed in delicate areas, such as when thinning bone over the facial nerve. As a general rule, always using the largest bur possible, which will reduce the chance of plunging a small bur into a critical structure. Irrigate frequently to avoid thermal injury to bone and surrounding critical structures (eg, nerves). Your nondominant hand will usually contain a suction-irrigator or, if irrigation is built into the drill, a plain suction. Drill in broad, smooth controlled strokes, rather than quick erratic strokes. Finally, avoid kinking of electric drill tubing, as airflow through the patent tube helps keep the drill cool.

Microdrill

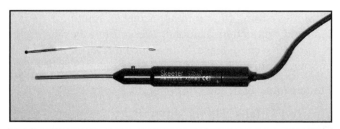

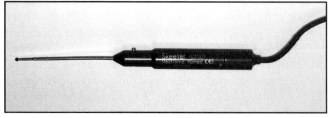

Aliases and Nicknames: Skeeter drill, Skeeter

Uses: Drilling through small, intricate regions of the temporal bone, such as the facial recess, stapes footplate, or when creating a cochleostomy for cochlear implantation.

Description: Bur (drill bit) has a proximal wire that is inserted through the distal end of the drill (bur aside in first image, bur installed in second image). Various bur sizes are available. Rotational speed is controlled with a foot pedal.

Tips and Pitfalls: Burs are nondisposable.

Miscellaneous Instruments

NIM (Nerve Integrity Monitor) Incrementing Probe, Prass Tip

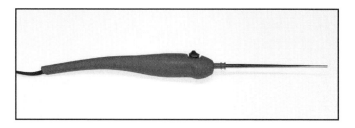

Aliases and Nicknames: NIM Prass probe

Uses: Stimulating the facial nerve for positive identification.

Description: Long needle attached to a handle with a switch. Depressing switch electrically stimulates the structure contacting the tip. The output of the stimulator may be varied. Connects to the Nerve Integrity Monitor (facial nerve monitor) console.

Dimensions: 24 cm long including tip

CHAPTER

Nasal and Sinus Surgery

Jae H. Lim and Greg E. Davis

CONTENTS

Cutting Instruments
Microdebrider (Straight, Curved)
Drill Bit Attachment for Microdebrider (Straight, Curved)
Sickle Knife
Turbinate Scissors (Straight, Curved Left, Curved Right)

Forceps
Takahashi Nasal Forceps
Backbiting Forceps
Straight Weil-Blakesley Forceps
45° Weil-Blakesley Forceps
Suction Straight (or 45°) Weil-Blakesley Forceps
Giraffe Sinus Forceps
Jansen-Middleton Septum Forceps
Bayonet Forceps

Wormald Malleable Instruments
Wormald Malleable Suction Curette
Wormald Malleable Suction Probe
Wormald Malleable Tool Bender

Miscellaneous Instruments
Nasal Speculum
Wormald Knot Pusher
Olive Tip Sinus Suction
Frazier Suction

Rigid Telescopes

0° Hopkins Telescope

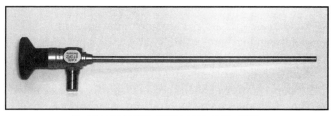

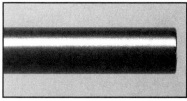

Aliases and Nicknames: 0° Hopkins endoscope, 0° Hopkins rod, 0° Hopkins rod lens, 0° rigid scope, 0° scope

Uses: Provides a magnified view of the operative field during endoscopic surgery.

Description: Straight rigid telescope. The image is carried through a series of lenses and glass rods in the shaft (hence the term "rod lens") and is not fiber-optic. The eyepiece (black, flared end in first image above) attaches to a high-definition camera (not pictured), which in turn is connected to a box connected to a high-definition display. The side adapter near the eyepiece attaches to a fiber-optic light source. The tip of the endoscope is aimed at the surgical field of interest. The image is then displayed on a high-definition monitor in real time.

Dimensions: Length and diameter vary depending on application.

Tips and Pitfalls: The 0° endoscope is used predominantly for the initiation of the maxillary antrostomy, the ethmoidectomy, and the sphenoidotomy. Avoid resting the tip directly on the drapes while the light source is on as this could cause a fire.

Notes

■ Rigid telescopes are used for many purposes in otolaryngology. For example, similar designs with longer shafts are used to obtain magnified images during direct laryngoscopy, bronchoscopy, and esophagoscopy. Narrower shafts are available for pediatric use.

■ The telescope is named after its inventor Harold Hopkins, a British physicist, not after Johns Hopkins University. The term "Hopkins" is a trademark of Karl-Storz; however, alternative brand scopes of a similar design are available.

■ When performing endoscopic sinus surgery, rigid telescopes may be placed within an irrigating sheath system. This allows the surgeon to clean the lens tip if it becomes covered with blood, maintaining visualization without removing the telescope from the nasal cavity. Several systems are available, including Endo-Scrub and Clearvision. Alternatively, one may use an antifog solution.

30° Hopkins Telescope

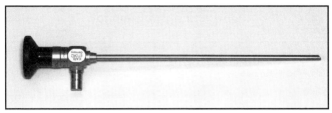

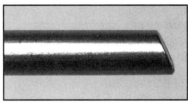

Aliases and Nicknames: 30° Hopkins endoscope, 30° Hopkins rod, 30° Hopkins rod lens, 30° rigid scope, 30° scope

Uses: Provides a magnified view of the operative field during endoscopic sinus surgery.

Description: Similar to 0° Hopkins telescope, but with an angled tip. The distal end of endoscope is aimed at the surgical field of interest at 30 degrees.

Dimensions: Varies

Tips and Pitfalls: The 30° endoscope is used mainly when clearing the ethmoid sinuses off the skull base, during frontal sinus surgery, or to complete the maxillary antrostomy and exploration. Angles of 45°, 70°, and more are also available for more advanced techniques.

Elevators, Rongeurs, and Curettes

Cottle Septum Elevator

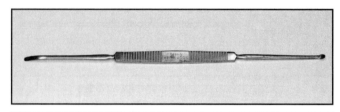

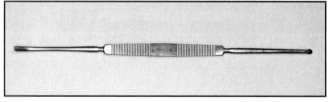

Aliases and Nicknames: Cottle elevator, Cottle

Uses: Elevating a mucosal flap off of bone or cartilage. Commonly used for septoplasty to raise the mucoperichondrial and mucoperiosteal flaps. Also may be used to lift the mucosa off the turbinate bone during submucosal inferior turbinate reduction or to raise a septal mucosal flap during cerebrospinal fluid (CSF) leak repair.

Description: Has sharp (right side in images above) and dull (left side in images above) dissecting ends to facilitate elevation of the flap.

Dimensions: 23 cm long

Tips and Pitfalls: Always keep the tip firmly on the bone or cartilage when elevating to reduce the chance of perforating the flap.

Gorney Suction Elevator

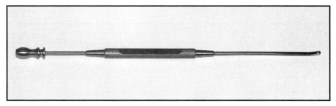

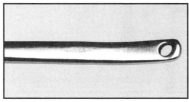

Aliases and Nicknames: Gorney suction, suction Gorney

Uses: Similar to Cottle septum elevator, but has the ability to provide local suction for improved visualization.

Description: The dissecting end, which is dull, has a suction port just proximal to the tip, allowing clearance of blood during dissection.

Dimensions: 21 cm long

Tips and Pitfalls: The amount of suction power can be controlled by sealing or unsealing the shaft suction port with an index finger or thumb. As with the Cottle septum elevator, keep the tip firmly on the bone or cartilage to reduce the chance of perforating the flap.

Straight Upbiting Kerrison Rongeur, Straight Downbiting Kerrison Rongeur

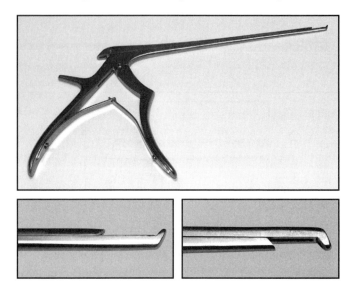

Aliases and Nicknames: Straight upbiter, straight down-biter. A similar version of this instrument is the Hajek-Kofler punch.

Uses: Used in endoscopic sinus surgery. For ethmoidectomy, used to cut ethmoid sinus bony septations. For sphenoid-otomy, used to enlarge the sphenoid os. Use is often immediately followed by the microdebrider or forceps to remove rongeured fragments of bone and mucosa.

Description: Contains two tip components that slide against one another, the longer of which has a hook on its distal end. The distal hook is either pointed up (upbiting; first and second images) or down (downbiting; third image). In the open position, there is space between the two sliding tips; this distance decreases as the handle is squeezed. In this manner, the tip can be opened and closed to grasp and cut bone.

Dimensions: 25 cm long

Tips and Pitfalls: The instrument should be inserted and withdrawn from the nose in a closed position to help minimize trauma to normal tissue. Steps for usage:

1. Insert the hooked tip above or below the bony ledge to be broken, then gently pull back toward yourself to be sure that the hook is engaged behind the bony ledge.
2. Next, squeeze the handle while continuing to gently pull back so that the nonhooked sliding tip moves forward to contact the hooked tip and cut the bone.
3. Do not pull away while you are breaking bone, as you may avulse excess tissue; rather, cut the bone and then gently release the tissue to leave it in place.
4. The cut bone and mucosa can then be removed with forceps or with the microdebrider.

Curved Upbiting Kerrison Rongeur

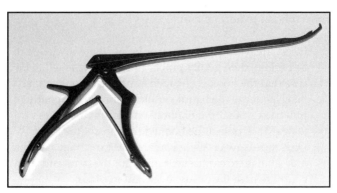

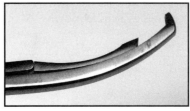

Aliases and Nicknames: Curved upbiter

Uses: Similar to the straight Kerrison rongeur with the added benefit of curved orientation. This allows removal of tissue and bony fragments in difficult to reach areas such as the frontal sinus region.

Description: Same as straight Kerrison rongeur, but with curved tip.

Dimensions: 25 cm long

Tips and Pitfalls: Same as straight Kerrison rongeur.

Note: For other septum elevators, periosteal elevators, and rongeurs, see pp. 269–286.

Sphenoid Punch

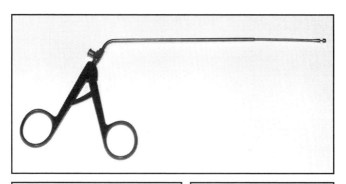

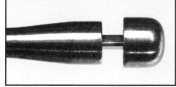
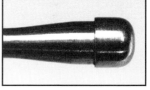

Uses: Sphenoidotomy during endoscopic sinus surgery.

Description: The dome-shaped distal end slides into sphenoid os while the proximal ledge anchors against bony edges of sphenoid os. Closeup images above depict open and closed positions.

Dimensions: 25 cm long

Tips and Pitfalls: Engage the instrument once the proximal ledge anchors the bony edge of sphenoid os. As the handles are squeezed, the dome-shaped end will retract and the bony edges will be fractured, thus widening the sphenoid os.

Antrum Curette (Straight, Curved)

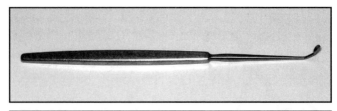

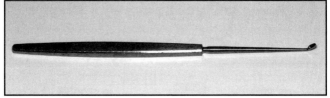

Aliases and Nicknames: Curette, straight curette, curved curette

Uses: Breaking apart bony partitions such as ethmoid cells during endoscopic sinus surgery.

Description: At the tip, curette has sharp edges that can dig into tissues and/or fracture bony partitions. Tips may have different angulations.

Dimensions: 20 cm long

Cutting Instruments

Microdebrider (Straight, Curved)

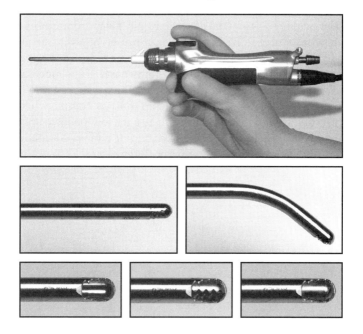

Aliases and Nicknames: Straight (or curved) debrider

Uses: Debriding tissue during endoscopic sinus surgery. The curved version is commonly used for frontal sinus surgery.

Description: The main workhorse during sinus surgery, this powered instrument has a rotary cutting tip that is used to shave tissue and thin bone. The neck is either straight (second image) or curved (third image) and is interchangeable. The microdebrider is connected to suction (via the metal ending at the top rear end of instrument in first image), which removes excess blood and tissue. The rotating action of the internal component of the tip is controlled with a foot pedal. Closeup images (fourth through sixth images) depict the rotary blades open, partly closed, and closed.

Dimensions: Powered handle (without tip) is 16 cm long

Tips and Pitfalls: The correct way to hold the microdebrider is depicted in the first image. Excess debridement can be avoided by a frequent "touch and come away" action. Remove foot from pedal *after* taking tip away from mucosa to avoid mucosal avulsion (mucosal preservation is a tenet of modern endoscopic sinus surgery). The debrider tip is sharp and can easily traumatize healthy nasal/sinus mucosa. When the tip is open, mucosa will tend to get sucked into it because of the suction. Thus, to avoid mucosal trauma when inserting/removing from the nose, use the foot pedal to spin the tip blades closed prior to insertion or removal (a mode can also be set to do this automatically).

Drill Bit Attachment for Microdebrider
(Straight, Curved)

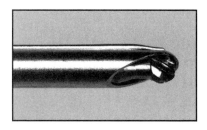

Aliases and Nicknames: Straight (or curved) drill

Uses: Drilling through bone during endoscopic sinus surgery.

Description: Straight or curved drill bit (bur) attachments for microdebrider. Cutting bur is pictured above. See microdebrider entry above for more details.

Tips and Pitfalls: A higher rpm (revolutions per minute) is used for drilling than for debriding. Irrigation is used to keep the drill bit and bone cool.

Sickle Knife

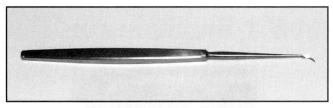

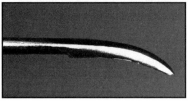

Uses: Uncinectomy during endoscopic sinus surgery, orbit decompression, endoscopic dacryocystorhinostomy.

Description: A sickle-shaped blade is at the tip that can penetrate nasal mucosa and thin bone.

Dimensions: 19 cm long

Tips and Pitfalls: The knife is used to penetrate the vertical portion of uncinate mucosa and bone to create a superior margin of the uncinectomy in the "swing door" technique for maxillary antrostomy.

Turbinate Scissors
(Straight, Curved Left, Curved Right)

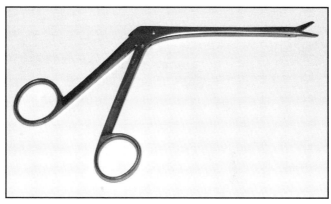

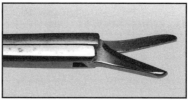

Aliases and Nicknames: Turb scissors

Uses: Inferior turbinate reduction, middle turbinate resection, concha bullosa resection.

Description: Pistol grip handle with a thin shaft. Tip contains scissor blades that allow for easy resection of inferior or middle turbinate during sinus surgery. Straight (pictured above), curved left, and curved right tips are available.

Dimensions: 19–20 cm long

Tips and Pitfalls: For any instruments with different types of tips, such as turbinate scissors to the right or left, know which type of tip you want before asking, and then ask for the proper specific instrument.

Forceps

Takahashi Nasal Forceps

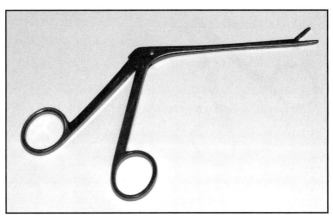

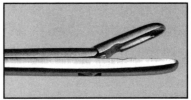

Aliases and Nicknames: Takahashi

Uses: Removal of free tissue fragments during endoscopic sinus surgery.

Description: Pistol grip handle with a thin shaft. Tips contain a cupped center. Tips do not have a sharp cutting action or a serrated edge. Also available with up-directed tips of various angles.

Dimensions: 18 cm long

Tips and Pitfalls: Used to grasp and remove tissue that has minimal remaining attachments. To sharply remove tissue, use the Weil-Blakesley forceps (see pp 144–146).

Backbiting Forceps

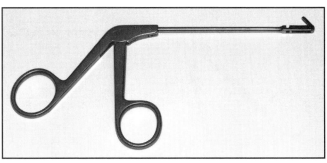

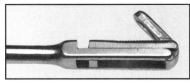

Aliases and Nicknames: Backbiter

Uses: Maxillary antrostomy during endoscopic sinus surgery.

Description: Pistol grip handle with a thin shaft. Tip includes a serrated base and a hinged rongeur. Opening the handles increases the angle between the serrated base and the hinged rongeur, whereas closing the handles decreases the angle to fracture or grasp tissue. In this manner, the tip opens and closes to engage and fracture the maxillary antrum and uncinate process for removal.

Dimensions: 19–20 cm long

Tips and Pitfalls: To engage the uncinate:

1. Open the handles fully to open the hinged distal tip.
2. Rotate the tip laterally and posteriorly around the uncinate process to engage it.
3. Rotate the instrument medially while gently pulling back toward yourself. This will bring the uncinate process medially into the nasal cavity.
4. In this position, the uncinate can then be fractured by squeezing the handles and closing the hinged tip.

Straight Weil-Blakesley Forceps

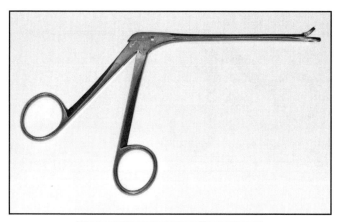

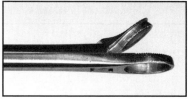

Aliases and Nicknames: Through-biter, "thru-cutting" forceps

Uses: Cuts through (hence the nickname) tissue and bony fragments for easy removal from the surgical field.

Description: Pistol grip handle with a thin shaft. Tip contains a punch-like jaw with a serrated edge that fractures tissue as the handles are squeezed together.

Dimensions: 19–20 cm long

Tips and Pitfalls: For grasping and removing tissue that is already nearly detached, use the Takahashi forceps instead.

45° Weil-Blakesley Forceps

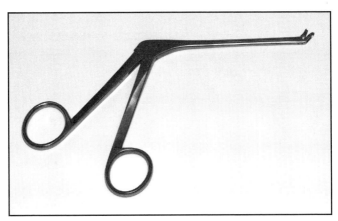

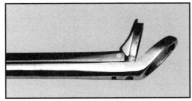

Aliases and Nicknames: 45° through cutter, 45° "thru-cutting" forceps

Uses: Uncinectomy, tissue removal. The sharply angled tip allows for removal of otherwise hard-to-reach soft tissue and/or bony fragments during endoscopic sinus surgery. See also straight Weil-Blakesley forceps.

Description: Similar to the straight Weil-Blakesley forceps, except that the tips are rotated upward at a 45° angle for improved reach in certain areas.

Dimensions: 19-20 cm long

Tips and Pitfalls: See straight Weil-Blakesley forceps (previous entry).

Suction Straight (or 45°) Weil-Blakesley Forceps

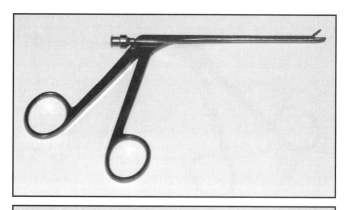

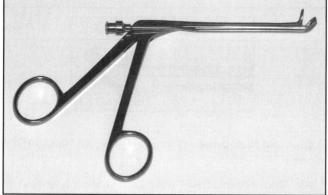

Uses: Similar to the standard Weil-Blakesley forceps, except with the capability of suctioning blood and debris from the surgical field for improved visualization.

Description: Similar design to standard Weil-Blakesley forceps, but with the addition of a suction tube that reaches the tip.

Dimensions: 17 cm long

Tips and Pitfalls: See straight Weil-Blakesley forceps (p. 144).

Giraffe Sinus Forceps

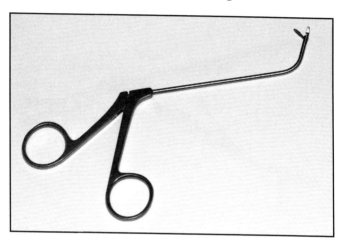

Aliases and Nicknames: Giraffe

Uses: Accessing the frontal sinus during frontal sinus surgery.

Description: Pistol grip handle with a thin shaft. The neck is long and angled. This allows one to grasp tissues in the far reaches of the frontal sinus. These are available with a variety of tip styles including through-cutting and grasping forceps.

Dimensions: 19–20 cm long

Jansen-Middleton Septum Forceps

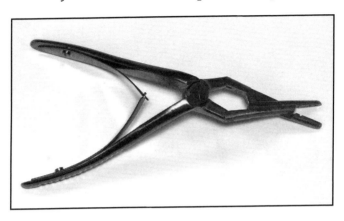

Aliases and Nicknames: Double action through-biting forceps

Uses: Removal of deviated bony septum and spurs.

Description: Double action forceps with tips that are able to remove bone.

Dimensions: 18 cm long

Tips and Pitfalls: Insert into nose while closed to minimize damaging adjacent tissue. Ensure tissue has been fully transected before removing the forceps from the nose to minimize tearing.

Bayonet Forceps

See p. 4.

Wormald Malleable Instruments

Wormald Malleable Suction Curette

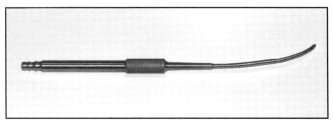

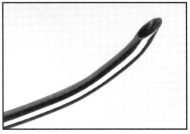

Uses: Curettage of hard-to-reach tissue during endoscopic sinus surgery. Curette tip allows removal of bony partitions and/or tissue.

Description: Curette tip with a malleable neck that can be bent to various angles to access hard-to-reach regions. Proximal end attaches to suction line.

Dimensions: 22 cm long

Tips and Pitfalls: This instrument can be very useful when trying to remove bony fragments and partitions of ethmoid cells along the skull base. The malleable neck should always be bent with the Wormald malleable tool bender (see p. 151) and not by hand, which could damage the instrument.

Wormald Malleable Suction Probe

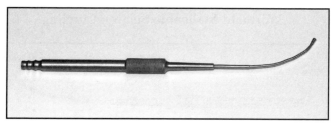

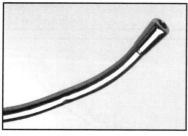

Uses: Suction and exploration of narrow regions during endoscopic sinus surgery, such as the frontal sinus or the floor of the maxillary sinus.

Description: Blunt suction tip with malleable neck that can be bent to various angles to access hard-to-reach regions. Proximal end attaches to suction line.

Dimensions: 21 cm long

Tips and Pitfalls: The malleable neck should always be bent with the Wormald malleable tool bender (see next entry) and not by hand, which could kink the shaft and damage the instrument.

Wormald Malleable Tool Bender

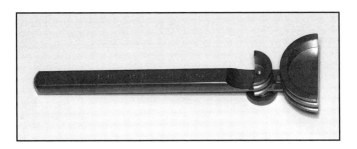

Uses: Bends the neck of Wormald malleable instruments to various angles.

Description: Straight handle/shaft. Distal end contains a bender consisting of small and large arcs.

Dimensions: 15 cm long

Tips and Pitfalls: The neck of the Wormald malleable instrument is inserted between the two arcs and bent to the desired angle. It is important to always use this tool to bend the Wormald instruments (rather than bending by hand) to minimize kinking of the malleable metal, which can damage the instruments.

Miscellaneous Instruments

Nasal Speculum

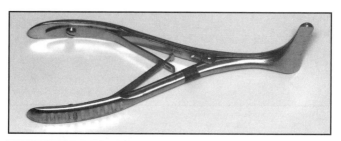

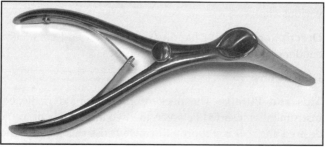

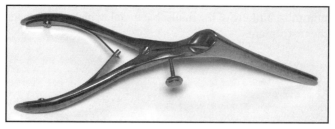

Uses: Visualizing the nasal cavity during nasal surgery.

Description: Spring-loaded handle with variable blade length. Some designs have a thumbscrew (second and third images, note variable locations) to lock the blade position.

Dimensions: Varies

Tips and Pitfalls: When performing septoplasty, may start with a shorter bladed speculum and switch to longer bladed speculum as the case progresses.

Wormald Knot Pusher

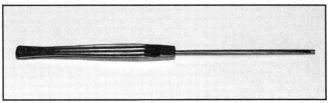

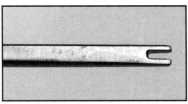

Uses: Notch at the distal end of the instrument is used to tie suture knots in the nasal cavity.

Description: Slim shaft with a small notch in the tip.

Dimensions: 20 cm long

Tips and Pitfalls: Can be used to suture the middle turbinate to the septum or to secure a fat plug during cerebrospinal fluid (CSF) leak repair.

Olive Tip Sinus Suction

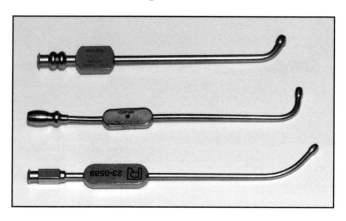

Aliases and Nicknames: Olive tip suction

Uses: Suctioning during endoscopic sinus surgery.

Description: The bulbous suction tip has smooth round edges and exists in various angles to allow evacuation and irrigation of debris and sinus contents. The proximal end is connected to a suction line.

Dimensions: 10-12 cm long (varies)

Tips and Pitfalls: These are especially useful for suctioning contents from the maxillary and frontal sinuses. A syringe filled with saline also may be attached for flushing.

Frazier Suction

See Frazier Suction, Baron Suction, p. 71.

CHAPTER

Laryngologic Surgery

Jack J. Liu,* Arun Sharma,* and
Tanya K. Meyer

CONTENTS

*equal contribution

Laryngoscope Accessories
Laryngoscope Suspension Systems
Fiber-Optic Light Carrier for Laryngoscope
Light Clip
Dual Chamber Light Carrier
Suction Tube for Laryngoscopy
Velvet-Eye Suction Tube for Laryngoscopy
Microlaryngeal Suction Tube
Lindholm Laryngeal Distending Forceps

Esophagoscopes
Rigid Esophagoscope

Esophagoscope Accessories
Velvet-Eye Suction for Esophagoscopy
Fiber-Optic Light Carrier for Esophagoscope

Rigid Hopkins Telescopes
0°, 30°, and 70° Hopkins Telescopes

Tracheotomy-Specific Instruments
Cricoid Hook
Tracheal Dilator

Microlaryngeal Instruments
Heart-Shaped Grasper (Right or Left)
Alligator Forceps (Straight, Curved Right, Curved Left)
Cup Forceps (Straight, Angled Up, Curved Left,
    Curved Right)
Laryngeal Scissors (Straight, Angled Up, Curved
    Left, Curved Right)
Ball Tip Probe (Straight or Angled)
Spatula
Laryngeal Sickle Knife
Laryngeal Knot Pusher

Thyroplasty Instruments
Long Elevator
Double-Ended Elevator
Window Template

Measuring Probe
Silastic Block Holder

Dilators and Miscellaneous Instruments
Jackson Laryngeal Dilator
Jackson Esophageal Dilator
Laser Platform Suction

Note: For bronchoscopes, see pp. 237–240.

Laryngoscopes

Lindholm Laryngoscope

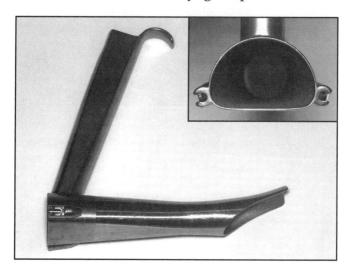

Note: For pediatric Lindholm laryngoscope, see pp. 232–234.

Aliases and Nicknames: Lindholm

Uses: Direct laryngoscopy and suspension laryngoscopy (with or without a microscope or telescope). A commonly used first-line laryngoscope due to wide exposure of the supraglottis, glottis, and hypopharynx.

Description: This laryngoscope is designed for the upper blade (flared distal superior tip) to engage the vallecula or hyoepiglottic ligament. The upper blade can be placed in an endolaryngeal manner, but doing so may cause some trauma. This scope has a large dome-shaped viewing window, large distal viewing window, and side ports for fiber-optic light carriers and oxygen carriers. The inferior cutout at the distal end gives more exposure to the posterior glottis and hypopharynx. It has a large flared distal superior tip to displace the epiglottis. Like most Storz laryngoscopes, the handle is at approximately 70° with a distal hook.

Dimensions: 39 mm proximal width, 18 mm distal width

Tips and Pitfalls: Laryngoscopes are traditionally held in the left hand. Begin on one side of the oral cavity using the laryngoscope to sweep the tongue laterally. Advance slowly. Make sure the vector of force suspends from the mandible and does not create a fulcrum against the front teeth. Manufacturer is Storz.

Steiner Laryngoscope

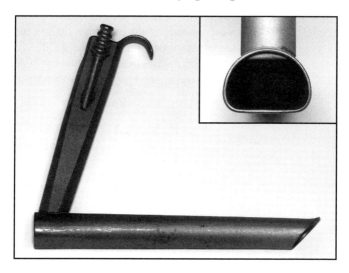

Aliases and Nicknames: Steiner

Uses: Suspension laryngoscopy for transoral laser surgery

Description: Half-dome viewing window, beveled distal tip, and an acute angle grip handle with finger hook. Right side contains a smoke evacuation port that connects to a suction line. It is coated with an antireflective coating.

Dimensions: 25 mm proximal width, 16 mm distal width. Similar designs available as well, including some with longer blades.

Tips and Pitfalls: A light clip is required for this laryngoscope. Be sure to take proper precautions for transoral laser surgery. Manufacturer is Storz.

Steiner Distending Operating Laryngoscope (Winged)

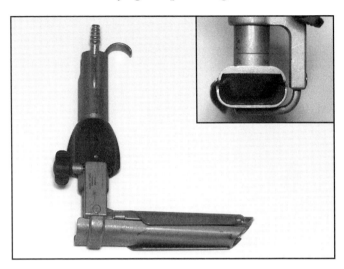

Aliases and Nicknames: Steiner set

Uses: Transoral laser surgery, useful for resection of large tumors or masses.

Description: Adjustable distal view, bilateral "wings" to prevent tongue/soft tissue from prolapsing between blades and obstructing the view, antireflective coating, channel at upper handle for suction attachment to evacuate smoke. Requires a light clip.

Dimensions: 14 cm long

Tips and Pitfalls: Close distending tips completely prior to laryngoscopy, check that tip adjustment is functional prior to use. Manufacturer is Storz.

Steiner Distending Operating Laryngoscope (Wingless)

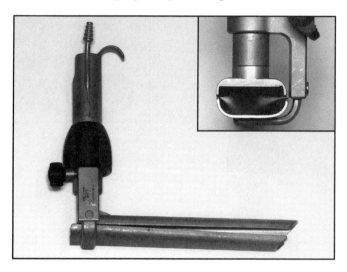

Aliases and Nicknames: Steiner set

Uses: Transoral laser surgery, useful in resection of large tumors or masses.

Description: Adjustable distal view, "wingless" model, antireflective coating, channel at upper handle for suction attachment to evacuate smoke.

Dimensions: 18 cm long

Tips and Pitfalls: Close distending tips completely prior to laryngoscopy and check that tip adjustment is functional. Manufacturer is Storz.

Dedo Laryngoscope

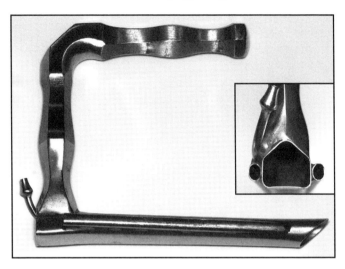

Aliases and Nicknames: Dedo

Uses: Direct laryngoscopy and suspension laryngoscopy. Large viewing window allows for visualization and instrumentation of endolarynx. Good first-line laryngoscope along with the Lindholm.

Description: Large "house-shaped" pentagonal viewing window, two side ports for dual chamber light source, oxygen or smoke evacuation port on the left. It has a beveled distal tip and right-angle grip handle typical of Pilling laryngoscopes.

Dimensions: 19 mm proximal width, 12 mm distal width

Tips and Pitfalls: This is compatible with the Lewy arm suspension system. Manufacturer is Pilling.

Ossoff-Pilling Laryngoscope

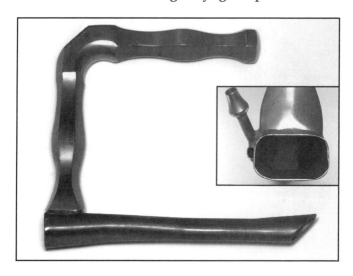

Aliases and Nicknames: Ossoff-Pilling, OP

Uses: Suspension laryngoscopy. Typically used for patients with difficult exposure of the larynx: trismus, limited neck extension, large tongue base, short/thick neck.

Description: Has a slim shaft that facilitates exposure in difficult cases. However, it gives a more limited view of the endolarynx compared to the Dedo or Lindholm. Right-angle handle with oxygen/suction port on the left. May have single or dual light chambers.

Dimensions: 26 mm anterior width, 8 mm distal width

Tips and Pitfalls: Smaller than the Dedo but may be better for difficult exposure cases. Compatible with the Lewy arm suspension system (see pp. 171–172). Manufacturer is Pilling.

Ossoff Male and Female Subglottiscope

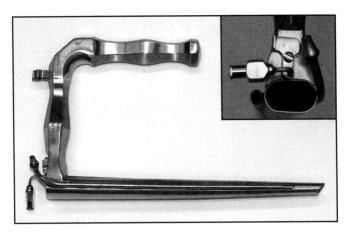

Aliases and Nicknames: Subglottiscope

Uses: Access to the subglottis for laser surgery with jet ventilation.

Description: Long narrow lumen for subglottic access. There is a port for the jet ventilation needle (seen inserted superior to viewing window in inset image), port for the light source (left of viewing window), and port for oxygen delivery or smoke evacuation (right of viewing window).

Dimensions: 21 mm proximal width, 9.5 mm distal width (male), 7.3 mm distal width (female)

Tips and Pitfalls: This scope is designed for the distal end to be placed through the vocal folds to expose the subglottis. Compatible with the Lewy arm suspension system (see pp. 171–172). Manufacturer is Pilling.

Weerda Distending Diverticuloscope

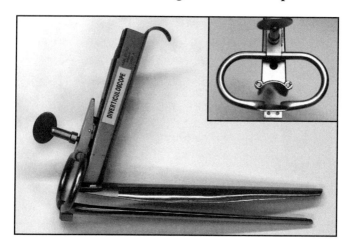

Aliases and Nicknames: Diverticuloscope

Uses: Zenker's diverticulectomy, cervical esophagoscopy.

Description: Bivalved laryngoscope with long adjustable blades. The blades distend vertically and also hinge open in a clamshell manner.

Dimensions: 40 mm proximal width, 27 mm distal width. 24 cm length.

Tips and Pitfalls: Adjust the two blades as needed for a good fit. For Zenker's diverticula, the posterior blade is inserted into the diverticulum and anterior blade into the native esophagus to expose the soft tissue bar between them so that it can be divided. Manufacturer is Storz.

Zeitels Universal Modular Glottiscope System

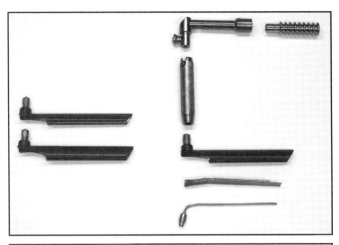

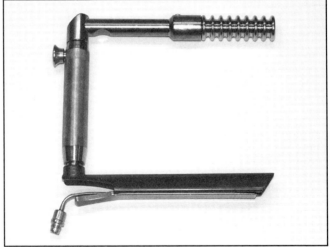

Aliases and Nicknames: Zeitels scope

Uses: Designed to be used for optimal visualization of the endolarynx (anterior commissure, false vocal folds, and true vocal folds, but not other parts of the supraglottis or hypopharynx). Due to the slim design, it is useful in difficult exposure cases. Blade is triangular shaped to conform to the internal shape of the thyroid cartilage and facilitate endolaryngeal exposure. This scope has a detachable baseplate that can facilitate intubation, bronchoscopy, or additional instrumentation (similar to a sliding Jackson laryngoscope, see next entry).

Description: Comes in three graduated sizes that attach to a universal handle. The baseplate slides into place as the "floor" of the laryngoscope and contains the light and oxygen/suction ports. The detachable baseplate can be removed once the scope is inserted to facilitate intubation, bronchoscopy, or additional instrumentation. The handle can be used with fulcrum suspension (see pp. 171–172) or with its own gallows suspension system (not pictured). The first image depicts a fully disassembled system. Note that alternative smaller and larger blades are pictured to the left. The second image depicts the assembled system.

Dimensions: Width of viewing tubes varies.

Tips and Pitfalls: Select the appropriate size/shape of viewing tube (ie, blade) for each particular patient; this can then be exchanged for a different tube to address any difficulties that are met. Manufacturer is Endocraft.

Sliding Jackson Laryngoscope

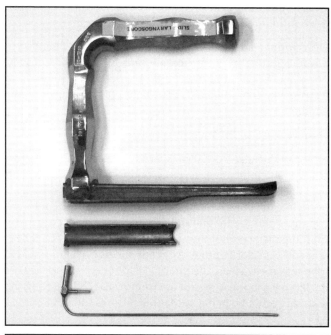

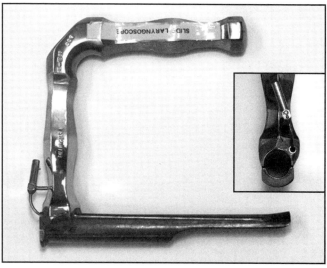

Aliases and Nicknames: Sliding Jackson

Uses: Intubation in difficult airway cases, direct laryngoscopy, introduction of rigid bronchoscopes.

Description: Laryngoscope with straight blade, similar to a Miller intubating laryngoscope but with better lighting. The floor of the laryngoscope will slide out to allow open instrumentation from below. The light port is attached to the handle.

Dimensions: 16 cm long

Tips and Pitfalls: The larynx can be exposed with the laryngoscope and intubation can be accomplished directly through the lumen of the scope. The advantages of this over the Miller or McIntosh "anesthesia" blades are that the Jackson laryngoscope holds the tongue and soft tissues of the mouth away from the distal end of the laryngoscope for better visualization and superior lighting. After advancing the endotracheal tube into the trachea, the inferior blade (floor/baseplate) of the laryngoscope can be slid out (removed) while leaving the endotracheal tube in place. Manufacturer is Pilling.

Laryngoscope Accessories

Laryngoscope Suspension Systems

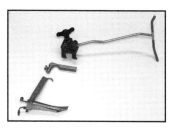
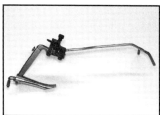
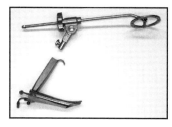
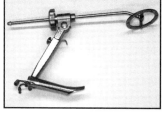

Aliases and Nicknames: Lewy suspension system, Lewy arm, Pilling suspension system (first and second images); Benjamin-Parsons suspension system, Storz suspension system (third and fourth images); Zeitels gallows suspension device (not pictured)

Uses: Hands-free suspension of laryngoscopes. This allows procedures to be performed with two hands under appropriate visualization.

Description: Two types of suspension systems are available:

■ *Fulcrum or rotation system:* This includes both devices pictured above. The suspension device attaches to the upper portion of the laryngoscope handle. Centrally, it includes a long arm (shaft). The distal end contains a bar-like platform (right side of first and second images) or circular platform (right side of third and fourth images) that is lowered onto a stable surface. This "suspends" the patient, thus holding the laryngoscope in position with some upward and rotational torque/force. Note that the pictured Lindholm laryngoscope requires an adapter to attach to the Lewy suspension system (first and second images). The system is called fulcrum or rotation because the platform acts as a point around which the remainder of the device pivots.

■ *Gallows system:* This system has a more appropriate upward vector of pull, but is less commonly available. The device may clamp onto the side of the bed, rather than resting on a stable surface (not pictured).

Dimensions: Varies

Tips and Pitfalls: Once an appropriate view is obtained with the laryngoscope of choice, the suspension system may be attached. It is often helpful to employ an assistant for this part. The distal end of a fulcrum suspension system (right side in above images) may be placed on towels, a Mayo stand, or another stable platform. Both devices pictured above have a knob that may be turned to increase the degree of suspension. The Lewy suspension system is for Pilling brand laryngoscopes, but will fit Storz scopes with an adapter. The Benjamin-Parsons suspension system fits Storz brand laryngoscopes. The suspension system can put significant pressure on teeth, gums, and the tongue, which can result in dental or oral trauma.

Fiber-Optic Light Carrier for Laryngoscope

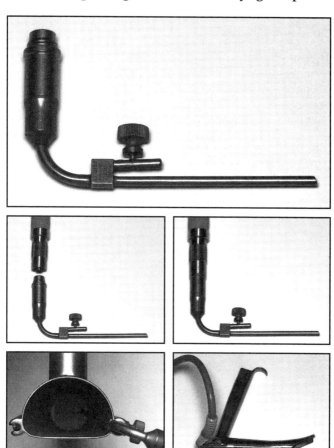

Aliases and Nicknames: Light carrier

Uses: Distal illumination for any laryngoscope with side light port (chamber).

Description: Long pole carries light through fiber optics, short pole with thumbscrew secures the carrier onto the laryngoscope. Proximal end screws onto fiber-optic cable to light source (second and third images). Fourth and fifth images depict the light carrier attached to a Lindholm laryngoscope.

Dimensions: Varies

Tips and Pitfalls: Light pole side is inserted into the laryngoscope lumen, conventionally placed on right side of laryngoscope (fourth and fifth image). As with any use of a fiber-optic light cable, be sure that the free end is not resting on the drapes when the light source is on, as this poses a fire hazard. With any airway or critical procedure, always test that your light source and setup are fully functioning well in advance, ideally before the patient arrives.

Light Clip

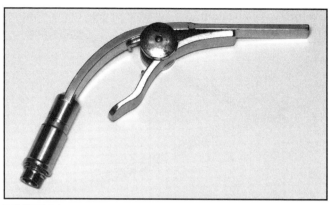

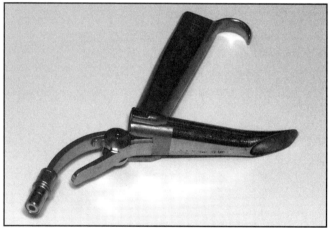

Uses: For proximal illumination and with laryngoscopes that do not contain light ports (chambers).

Description: Rectangular light window. Contains a bottom plate connected to an internal spring to maintain closing tension. Proximal end screws onto fiber-optic cable to light source (not depicted in images). Second image shows clip attached to a pediatric Lindholm laryngoscope.

Dimensions: Varies

Tips and Pitfalls: Depress the bottom plate to open the clip. Clip to opposite side of oxygen port if one is present. Obstructs visualization to a variable degree depending on laryngoscope size.

Dual Chamber Light Carrier

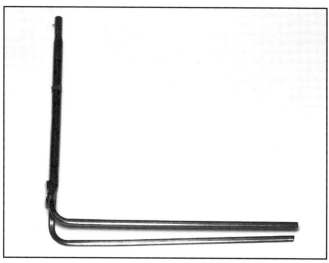

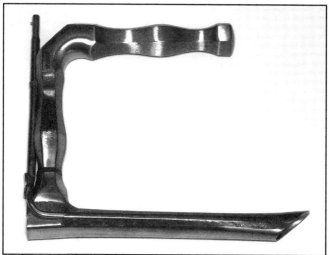

Aliases and Nicknames: Light carrier

Uses: Distal illumination for Ossoff-Pilling and Dedo laryngoscopes.

Description: Proximal end forks into two light poles. Proximal end screws onto fiber-optic cable (with single turn) to light source.

Dimensions: Varies

Tips and Pitfalls: Be sure cable to light source is inserted completely into the proximal end of the dual chamber light carrier, otherwise may result in poor illumination.

Suction Tube for Laryngoscopy

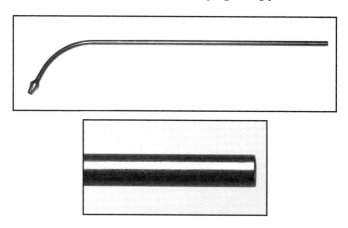

Aliases and Nicknames: Suction

Uses: Suction of blood and oral secretions.

Description: Single suction hole at distal tip, long shaft, curved proximal end for easy grip.

Dimensions: ~25 cm long (varies)

Tips and Pitfalls: Not appropriate for directly suctioning on vocal folds, as it may cause trauma. Instead, use the velvet-eye suction or microlaryngeal suction (see next two entries).

Velvet-Eye Suction Tube for Laryngoscopy

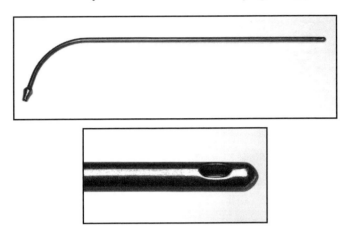

Aliases and Nicknames: Velvet tip suction, velvet tip

Uses: Suction of blood and oral secretions including in more delicate areas.

Description: Two side suction holes near tip, distal tip is dome shaped and not patent. Long shaft, curved proximal end for easy grip.

Dimensions: ~25 cm long (varies)

Tips and Pitfalls: Velvet eye side holes reduce suction-related trauma to vocal folds.

Microlaryngeal Suction Tube

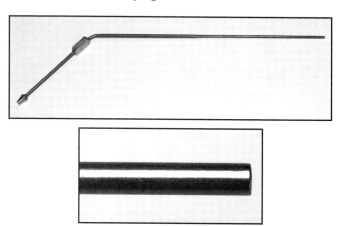

Aliases and Nicknames: Fine-tip suction, microsuction

Uses: Suctioning on laryngeal structures.

Description: Fine tip with single suction hole at distal end. Long shaft with proximal bend, thumb port for suction control.

Dimensions: ~31 cm long (varies)

Tips and Pitfalls: Release thumb port while suctioning on vocal folds to avoid trauma.

Lindholm Laryngeal Distending Forceps

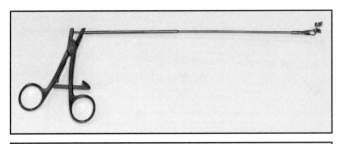

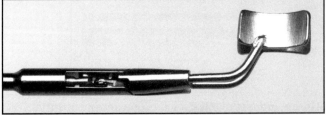

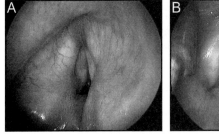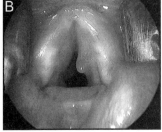

Endoscopic photos courtesy of Andrew F. Inglis, MD

Aliases and Nicknames: Laryngeal spreaders

Uses: Spreading (abducting) the false vocal folds to improve visualization of the true vocal folds.

Description: Pistol-grip handle with ratcheting mechanism, distal ends with gently curved rectangular blades designed to fit over the false vocal folds into the ventricles. As the handles are squeezed/ratcheted, the blades spread apart.

Tips and Pitfalls: Guide each blade over the false vocal folds before gently spreading. The dramatic improvement in visualization can be seen in the above endoscopic views of a glottis before (A) and after (B) use of the forceps. In the latter image (B) small subglottic cysts are revealed.

Esophagoscopes

Note: For pediatric rigid esophagoscope see pp. 241–243.

Rigid Esophagoscope

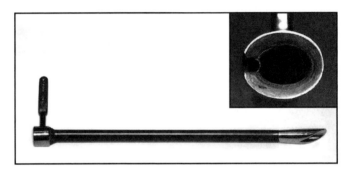

Aliases and Nicknames: Esophagoscope

Uses: Direct, rigid esophagoscopy and removal of esophageal foreign bodies (see also pp. 244–246).

Description: Oval proximal viewing window, side light carrier port (see also p. 186), blunted and beveled distal tip. The proximal fin-like extension is for attaching an optional handle.

Dimensions: ~30–50 cm long (varies; select appropriate size for each patient)

Tips and Pitfalls: Hold esophagoscope handle with longer distal lip facing anteriorly. Stabilize esophagoscope with right thumb while advancing. Once esophagus is entered, advance slowly under direct vision. Excessive force could result in perforating the esophageal wall.

Esophagoscope Accessories

Velvet-Eye Suction Tube for Esophagoscopy

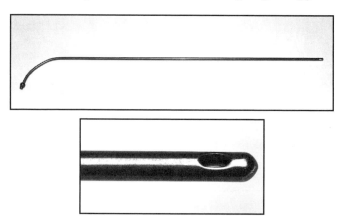

Aliases and Nicknames: See p. 180.

Uses: Suction for esophagoscopy

Description: Same as velvet-eye suction for laryngoscopy but longer.

Dimensions: ~48–67 cm long (varies)

Tips and Pitfalls: Select appropriate length to work with the paired esophagoscope well in advance, ideally before the patient arrives in the room. Test that the suction will fit and reach through the esophagoscope. This is especially critical with long adult or small pediatric esophagoscopes.

Fiber-Optic Light Carrier for Esophagoscope

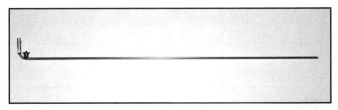

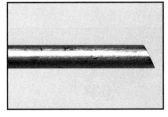
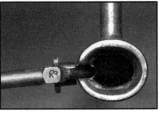

Aliases and Nicknames: Light carrier

Uses: Distal illumination during esophagoscopy.

Description: Long shaft, beveled tip, secures to esophago-scope (third image) with a thumb screw.

Dimensions: 43 cm long (varies)

Tips and Pitfalls: Choose appropriate length for paired esophagoscope.

Rigid Hopkins Telescopes

0°, 30°, and 70° Hopkins Telescopes

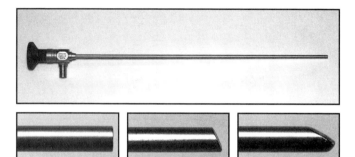

Alias and Nickname: 0° (or 30° or 70°) Hopkins endoscope, Hopkins rod, Hopkins rod lens, rigid telescope, rigid scope, scope

Uses: Provides a magnified view of the operative field during direct laryngoscopy, esophogoscopy, and bronchoscopy. 30° and 70° telescopes are helpful for viewing areas that are otherwise difficult to see, such as the laryngeal ventricles, anterior commissure, and subglottis.

Description: Proximal viewing window (black flared end at left of first image) connects to a camera that is then connected to a video monitor. Fiber-optic light cable secures with easy pop-in lock or via screwing mechanism to the proximal side port.

Dimensions: Varies; select appropriate length for paired laryngoscope, bronchoscope, or esophagoscope.

Tips and Pitfalls: Peer through viewing window prior to case to check telescope integrity. Handle the scopes carefully and do not bend them at all, as doing so can easily result in damage. For more information about Hopkins rigid telescopes see pp. 127–129.

Tracheotomy-Specific Instruments

Cricoid Hook

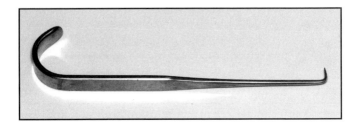

Aliases and Nicknames: Crich or cric (both pronounced "crike") hook

Uses: When performing a tracheotomy, a cricoid hook can be placed inferior to the cricoid and used to pull the trachea superiorly and anteriorly to improve exposure and access to the trachea.

Description: Single hook with a broad curved handle. Hook can be round or at a 90-degree angle. Tip of hook may be blunt or sharp.

Dimensions: ~14 cm long (varies)

Tips and Pitfalls: This instrument must be present whenever a tracheotomy is performed. The cricoid hook must remain in place until the tracheotomy is completed and correct placement of the tracheotomy tube confirmed by return of CO_2. If the hook is removed prematurely, it can be difficult to re-establish the airway.

Tracheal Dilator

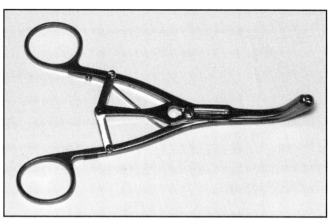

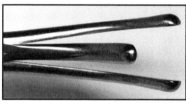

Aliases and Nicknames: Tracheal spreader, "trach" spreader, Laborde tracheal dilator (three prongs, as pictured), Trousseau tracheal dilator (two prongs, not pictured)

Uses: Widening the tracheal incision while performing tracheotomy.

Description: Three-pronged dilator with tines that open (second image) as the handles are squeezed. A two-pronged dilator is also available.

Dimensions: ~15 cm long

Tips and Pitfalls: Should be present whenever a tracheotomy may be performed.

Microlaryngeal Instruments

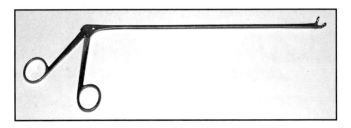

Note: All microlaryngeal forceps have a similar pistol-grip handle and long shaft, as depicted in image above. Tips only are depicted below.

Heart-Shaped Grasper (Right or Left)

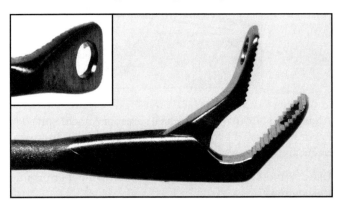

Aliases and Nicknames: Triangle-shaped grasper

Uses: Grasping and retracting tissue during laryngeal surgery.

Description: Grasper either angles to the right or left. The tips are triangular shaped with the broader part distal (see inset image of the tip viewed from below).

Tips and Pitfalls: This grasper can be used to gently grasp and manipulate tissue. Other laryngeal instruments can then be used simultaneously to further manipulate or excise tissue. Avoid excessive trauma to tissue when using the grasper.

Alligator Forceps (Straight, Curved Right, Curved Left)

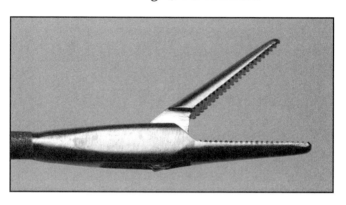

Uses: Grasping tissue during laryngeal surgery.

Description: Forceps with alligator teeth–like jaws.

Tips and Pitfalls: Avoid excessive trauma to tissue when using these forceps.

Cup Forceps (Straight, Angled Up, Curved Left, Curved Right)

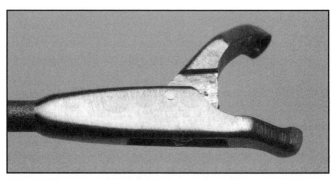

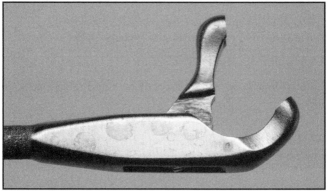

Aliases and Nicknames: Cups

Uses: Taking biopsies or removing tissue.

Description: Forceps tips are shaped like cups. Cup edges are sharp. Depicted above are curved left (first image) and angled up (second image) forceps.

Tips and Pitfalls: After grasping the tissue with these forceps while taking a biopsy, give a quick but gentle pull in order to avulse a small amount of tissue.

Laryngeal Scissors (Straight, Angled Up, Curved Left, Curved Right)

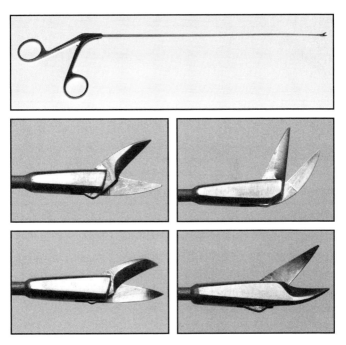

Uses: Cutting tissue in or near the larynx.

Description: Small, sharp microscissors, available with blades at multiple angles (second through fifth images) for easy access.

Ball Tip Probe (Straight or Angled)

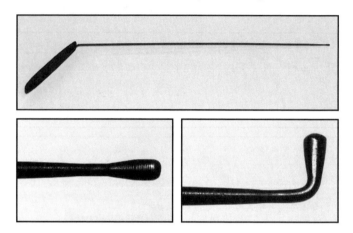

Uses: Palpating vocal folds gently for pathology such as scar, sulcus, nodules, and cysts.

Description: Small, blunt probe with a flared rounded tip that can be straight (second image) or at a 90° angle (third image). Handle is a broad plate (on left in first image).

Spatula

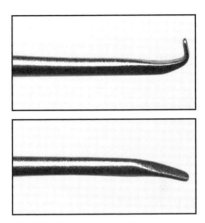

Aliases and Nicknames: Probe, elevator

Uses: Elevating tissue or flaps.

Description: Microlaryngeal instrument with blunt, tapered end available with variable amounts of curvature (eg, first versus second image).

Laryngeal Sickle Knife

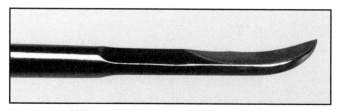

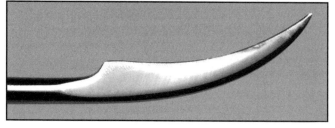

Aliases and Nicknames: Sickle knife, Blitzer blade

Uses: Fine cutting during laryngeal microsurgery (eg, incising the epithelium of the vocal fold to remove a benign lesion).

Description: Sickle-shape knife with a fine, nonserrated blade and fine tip.

Tips and Pitfalls: Be careful inserting and removing the sickle knife as it is very sharp and can easily damage tissue or the endotracheal tube. Make sure that it is guided into the laryngoscope by the scrub nurse/tech during microlaryngoscopy to avoid damage to the lips or face.

Laryngeal Knot Pusher

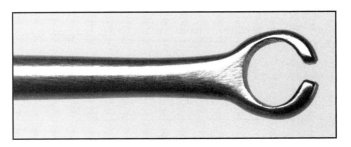

Uses: Manipulating suture and knots during microlaryngeal surgery.

Description: Tip contains a small, open loop that can be hooked around suture material for manipulation.

Thyroplasty Instruments

Note: The following instruments are from the Netterville thyroplasty set.

Long Elevator

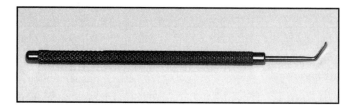

Uses: Elevating inner perichondrium from thyroid cartilage during thyroplasty.

Description: Knurled handle with a flat tip that is at an obtuse angle from the shaft.

Dimensions: 25 cm long

Double-Ended Elevator

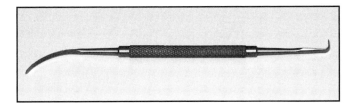

Uses: Elevating inner perichodrium from thyroid cartilage or other tissue during thyroplasty.

Description: Shaft contains knurled handle. Double-ended elevator with one end at a right angle and the other gently curved.

Dimensions: 17 cm long

Window Template

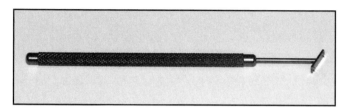

Uses: Used to help determine sizing of window in the thyroid cartilage during thyroplasty.

Description: Knurled handle with a flat rectangle at its distal end at an angle from the shaft. The angle facilitates holding the rectangular template flat against the thyroid cartilage. Rectangular template contains pointed studs near the four corners.

Dimensions: 16 cm long. Distal rectangular template measures 9 mm × 13 mm.

Tips and Pitfalls: Electrocautery applied to the handle will produce cautery marks at the points of contact with the studs. This allows marking of the window.

Measuring Probe

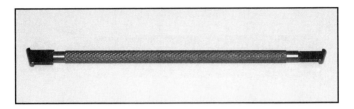

Uses: Determining amount of medialization in thyroplasty.

Description: Knurled central handle with two flared, rect-angular ends at angles from the shaft. The ends contain ruler markings. Larger end used for male patients and smaller end used for female patients.

Dimensions: 17 cm long

Silastic Block Holder

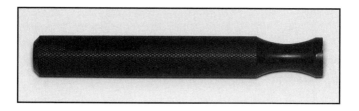

Uses: Silastic thyroplasty implant is placed in the holder to stabilize it during carving.

Description: Handled instrument with a distal end designed to snugly hold the silastic block.

Dimensions: 14 cm long

Dilators and Miscellaneous Instruments

Jackson Laryngeal Dilator

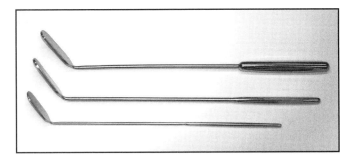

Aliases and Nicknames: Laryngeal dilator, Jackson tracheal dilator

Uses: Performing laryngeal dilation, often for stenosis.

Description: Handled instrument that resembles a golf club. The handle is the flat, short angled portion (left part of image). The distal end is flared and is used for dilation (right part of image).

Dimensions: ~30 cm long (varies). Tip ranges from 10 to 44 French based on the diameter of the dilating end.

Tips and Pitfalls: Despite looking like a golf club, the part that resembles the club head is actually the handle and the part that resembles the club grip is actually the dilator. In this respect, it is held like an upside-down golf club. Start with a small dilator and upsize sequentially until the desired degree of dilation is achieved.

Jackson Esophageal Dilator

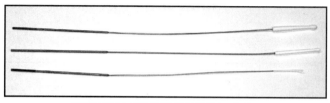

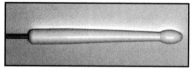

Aliases and Nicknames: Esophageal dilator

Uses: Performing esophageal dilation, such as for stenosis.

Description: Handled instrument with extremely long shaft. Contains a plastic tip with a distal flare that varies in size.

Dimensions: ~30 cm long (varies). Dilating tip ranges from 8 to 44 French.

Tips and Pitfalls: Start with a small dilator and upsize sequentially until the desired degree of dilation is achieved.

Laser Platform Suction

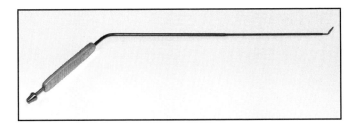

Aliases and Nicknames: Laser platform

Uses: Protecting tissues distal to the area of lasering.

Description: Broad handle with a bend in the proximal shaft. Tip contains a platform for protecting tissue. The distal end of platform usually contains a suction hole.

Dimensions: 32 cm long

Tips and Pitfalls: Placed just distal to the tissue where lasering will be applied. Tissue more distal to the platform is thus protected.

CHAPTER

Pediatric Otolaryngologic Surgery

Karthik Balakrishnan and Kathleen C. Y. Sie

CONTENTS

Palate and Miscellaneous Oral Instruments
Palate Scissors
Hockey Stick Elevator
Double-Ended Palate Elevator
Mitchell Trimmer
Salyer Cleft Palate Elevator, 90°
Single-Ended Palate Elevator, 90°
Single-Ended Palate Elevator, Hooked
Grooved Director

Pediatric Airway and Endoscopic Instruments
Fiber-Optic Light Carrier
Light Clip
Pediatric Lindholm Laryngoscope
Parsons Laryngoscope
Rigid Bronchoscope
Rigid Esophagoscope
Endoscopic Foreign Body Forceps

Myringotomy
Myringotomy Knife

Mouth Retractors (Mouth Gags)

McIvor Retractor

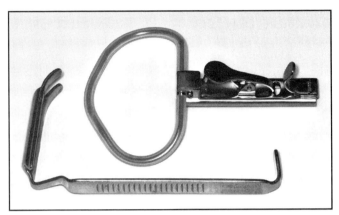

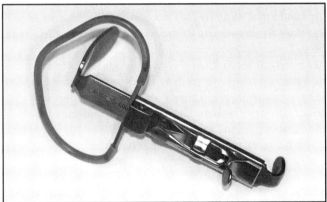

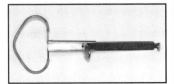
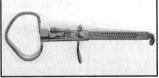

Aliases and Nicknames: McIvor mouth gag, McIvor

Uses: Props mouth open and depresses tongue for oral or transoral surgery. Commonly used for tonsillectomy and other operations in which the surgeon is at the head of the bed looking into the oral cavity and pharynx.

Description: Distinguished by closed, rounded loop of metal, often with rubberized coating to protect teeth. The retractor consists of two components, the main body (upper right in first image above) and the blade (bottom left in first image). The main body has a ratcheting mechanism that allows insertion of blades of various shapes and sizes. Blade shapes include flat (depicted in second through fourth images) and grooved (depicted in first image), with the grooved blades designed to accommodate and retract an oral endotracheal tube. The end opposite the metal loop contains a hook used for suspension (bottom right in second image).

Dimensions: Varies

Tips and Pitfalls: Flat blades typically are used in cases requiring clear visualization of deeper structures such as the tongue base. These blades are most easily used in combination with nasotracheal intubation. Grooved blades, in contrast, are designed to sit over orotracheal tubes (either straight or RAE tubes), for example, in tonsillectomy/adenoidectomy. The endotracheal tube should be taped to the midline of the chin to facilitate placement of the retractor blade. Correct assembly of the retractor is key to proper function.

Assembly and Placement of the McIvor Retractor:

1. Orient the loop of the main body so that its apex points toward you.
2. Hold the blade pointing toward the patient and insert it into the ratcheting body of the retractor, blade end first.
3. Depress the lever in the middle of the instrument and slide the blade forward, toward the closed loop.
4. The blade should end up near the loop, with the blade and depressed end of the loop pointing the same way.
5. With the blade completely inserted into the body of the retractor, insert the retractor into the mouth with the

loop toward the patient's head and the hook toward the feet.

6. Making sure that the tongue is midline and not pinched between blade and teeth, gently insert the blade until the bent tip of the loop is against the palate just posterior to the anterior maxillary teeth. Take care not to pinch the lip or compress the orotracheal tube, if present.

7. Once in place, the retractor can be ratcheted open to achieve the desired exposure.

8. If the tongue slips off the midline, you may need to reposition it with a blunt instrument or release ratcheting (press the lever in the middle of the instrument) and start over.

9. The hooked end can be suspended from a Mayo stand, towel roll, or other structure to further improve exposure.

Notes on Intraoperative Usage:

▨ If the patient begins to buck or cough while the retractor is open and suspended, the retractor should be released from suspension and partially closed. Otherwise, cervical spine injury may result if the Mayo stand is moved relative to the patient.

▨ While operating, take care that the blade does not come into contact with any cautery, as the metal may conduct heat and cause oral and lip burns.

Removal of the McIvor Retractor:

1. Communicate with the anesthesiologist, as retractor removal can be associated with inadvertent extubation.

2. Release retractor from suspension.

3. Depress the lever to return the blade to the original position. This will allow the mouth to close.

4. While securing the endotracheal tube, remove the retractor from the mouth.

Crowe-Davis Retractor

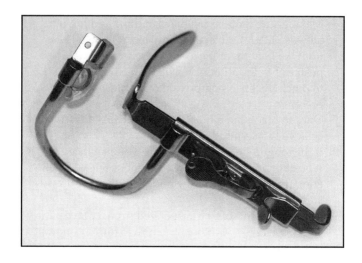

Aliases and Nicknames: Crowe-Davis mouth gag, Crowe-Davis

Uses: Similar to the McIvor retractor. Preferred by some surgeons over the McIvor due to larger area of metal loop, allowing more working space.

Description: Unlike McIvor retractor, this instrument has an incomplete metal loop with two rubberized tooth hooks designed to accommodate and protect the anterior maxillary teeth. The blades and ratcheting mechanism are the same as those of the McIvor.

Dimensions: Varies

Tips and Pitfalls: Assembly and setup is similar to the McIvor retractor. Ensure that the rubberized tooth hooks on the metal loop point in the same direction as the retractor blade. Insert and open the retractor in the same manner as the McIvor, making sure that the tooth hooks sit only on the teeth and do not pinch the upper lip. Remove the retractor in the same manner as the McIvor.

Dingman Retractor

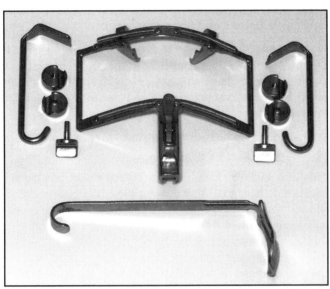

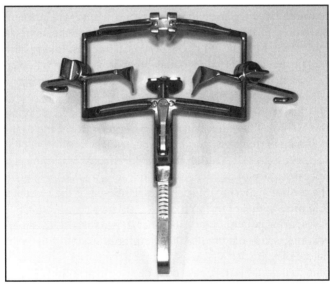

Aliases and Nicknames: Dingman mouth gag, Dingman

Uses: Oropharyngeal and palate surgery (eg, cleft palate repair, palatoplasty, and pharyngoplasty).

Description: Similar to the McIvor in its choice of blades, the use of a ratchet mechanism, and the use of suspension. Distinguished by large square frame with sliding tooth/lip hooks and cheek retractors. It also has springs on the flat upper and lower frame bars to secure suture tails.

Dimensions: Frame is 13 cm long and ~7.5 cm wide. Blades of different sizes are available.

Tips and Pitfalls: Each cheek retractor blade is attached to one side bar of the frame using the compression screws shown. The side bar of the frame fits into the groove of one half-screw, while the cheek retractor fits into the groove of the other half-screw. Use the thumbscrew to tighten the two half-screws against each other to secure the cheek retractor to the frame. It may be beneficial to assemble the cheek retractors such that the thumbscrews face away from the surgeon to minimize the chance that suture tails will tangle in them. Assembly of the frame and ratcheting blade is the same as that of the McIvor and Crowe-Davis retractors, taking care that the blade points in the same direction as the tooth hooks. Be sure that the tooth hooks are centered on the upper frame bar between the springs.

Insert the assembled retractor in a manner similar to the McIvor. Take care that the two depressions in the tooth hooks sit on the teeth and lip, respectively. Once the ratchet has been opened, position the cheek retractor blades on the buccal surface of each cheek and retract laterally to achieve the desired exposure on each side. Removal of the retractor is similar to that of the McIvor.

During palate surgery and pharyngeal surgery, the small working space may require that multiple sutures be placed before they are tied. Use the springs on the frame of the Dingman to hold the suture tails out of the surgeon's line of sight and to prevent tangling between suture tails.

Adenotonsillectomy Instruments

Adenoid Curette

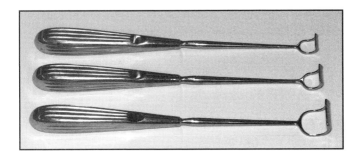

Uses: "Cold" (noncautery) transoral removal of adenoid tissue.

Description: Robust, grooved handle with long, narrow neck and curved metal loop at tip. Distal end of metal loop has a straight, flat edge.

Dimensions: 20–22 cm long

Tips and Pitfalls: Anterior retraction of the palate with a red rubber catheter inserted through the nose and looped out the mouth may make curette placement easier. Visualize the nasopharynx via the mouth using a mirror and headlight, and select a curette wide enough to cover the adenoid pad but narrow enough to avoid injury to the Eustachian tube tori. In general, the appropriate curette width can be estimated by the combined width of the two central incisors. Insert the curette with the distal end of the curve toward the palate in the midline. Carefully pass it into the nasopharynx and set it at the superior aspect of the adenoid pad, at the base of the vomer between the Eustachian tube tori on either side. Take care to stay against the posterior nasopharynx to avoid trauma to the choanae. Hold the grooved handle in one hand and the narrow neck in the other. Using the hand on the neck as a fulcrum, firmly sweep the curette inferiorly so that the sharp curette tip scrapes the adenoid tissue off the firm posterior nasopharyngeal wall. Stop curetting just cephalad to the margin of the soft palate. Remove the curette and the detached adenoid tissue, taking care not to let it fall toward the larynx to avoid aspiration. Use the mirror and a suction to examine the nasopharynx for any residual adenoid tissue, and achieve hemostasis using cautery or packing.

Choanal Curette

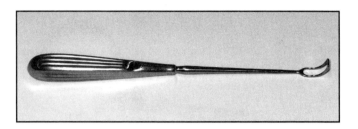

Uses: "Cold" (noncautery) transoral removal of adenoid tissue that protrudes from the nasopharynx into or through the posterior choanae.

Description: Similar to adenoid curette but with narrower tip.

Dimensions: 22 cm long

Tips and Pitfalls: Use in a manner similar to adenoid curette except that this curette typically is placed in a paramedian position. Take care not to catch the posterior end on the inferior turbinate, as this can cause troublesome bleeding.

St. Clair Forceps

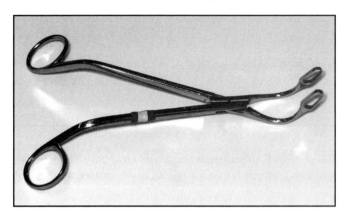

Aliases and Nicknames: St. Clair-Thompson adenoid forceps, St. Clair adenoid forceps

Uses: Transoral removal of adenoid tissue. Often used to remove residual adenoid fragments after the adenoid curette has been used.

Description: S-curved forceps with ring-shaped tips at the distal end of each tine.

Dimensions: 19 cm long

Tips and Pitfalls: The St. Clair forceps are designed to pass through the mouth and around the posterior edge of the soft palate, curving into the nasopharynx. Use it with one hand while visualizing the nasopharynx with a mirror in the other hand in order to precisely remove any significant areas of residual adenoid tissue. The rings will meet, biting the soft adenoid tissue and detaching it.

Laryngeal Mirror

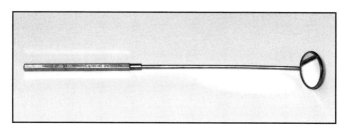

Aliases and Nicknames: Dental mirror, adenoid mirror, mirror

Uses: Intraoperative transoral examination of the nasopharynx and posterior choanae. Visualization of these areas during removal of adenoid tissue and during procedures involving the choanae. Clinic examination of the hypopharynx, larynx, and parts of the oral cavity.

Description: A small, round mirror angled at the end of a narrow handle and shaft.

Dimensions: 17 cm long, diameter of mirror varies

Tips and Pitfalls: Before insertion into the mouth, be sure to either warm the mirror or coat it with a thin layer of defogger solution to minimize fogging. pHisohex skin cleanser also works well for this purpose. When using the mirror, it may require some practice to become oriented to the inverted view of the nasopharynx and choanae. Rotate the handle slightly to examine different areas within the nasopharynx. Retraction of the soft palate will facilitate visualization of the nasopharynx. Larger mirrors typically offer the best view.

Fischer Knife

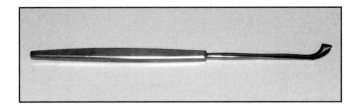

Aliases and Nicknames: Cold knife

Uses: "Cold" (noncautery) extracapsular removal of tonsils.

Description: Long, narrow handle with hockey stick-shaped, serrated blade. Blade is dull in order to allow dissecting (ie, it is not sharp for cutting).

Dimensions: 21 cm long

Tips and Pitfalls: Once the surgeon has defined the plane between the tonsillar capsule and the tonsillar fossa/superior constrictor muscle, this knife is useful in further dissection. Despite its name, this instrument is designed to be used for blunt dissection and not incising. As the surgeon separates the fossa away from the capsule, the two are held together by fibers of fascia. The serrations on the blade are not used to saw at these fibers. Rather, the blade is held perpendicular to the long axis of the tonsil and used to gently push the superior constrictor and its overlying fascia off the tonsil capsule. The serrations face the capsule and delicately strip off the fascial fibers. The key is to be in the correct plane.

Hurd Tonsil Dissector and Pillar Retractor

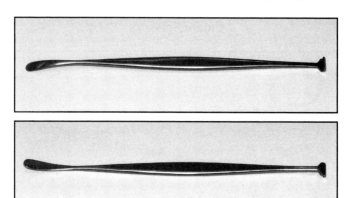

Aliases and Nicknames: Hurd retractor, Pillar retractor, Hurd

Uses: Transoral visualization of the tonsillar fossae.

Description: Long, narrow handle with one rounded spatula tip ("dissector"; on left in above images) and one broad, hooked tip ("pillar retractor"; on right in above images).

Dimensions: 21 cm long

Tips and Pitfalls: Very useful in tonsillectomy, particularly when examining the tonsillar fossa for bleeding sources after the tonsil is removed. The spatulated end is useful for pushing the superior end of the anterior tonsillar pillar superolaterally to expose the region of the superior pole. The hooked end may be used to retract the midpoint of the anterior pillar laterally to expose the fossa, but note that the hook can tear the mucosa of the pillar. The hook is also useful to visualize the inferior pole of the fossa: place the hook flat on the inferior portion of the posterior pillar and push it toward the midline to expose the inferior pole.

Note: For other frequently used adenotonsillectomy instruments, see Bovie electrocautery (p. 51), suction Bovie electrocautery (p. 52), and Allis tissue forceps (p. 15).

Palate and Miscellaneous Oral Instruments

Palate Scissors

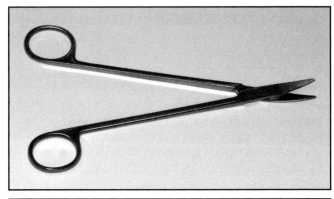

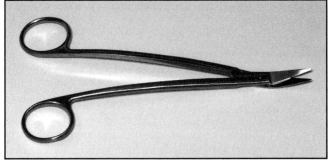

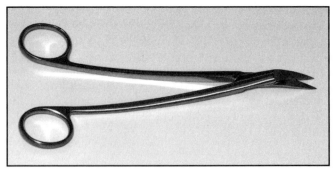

Aliases and Nicknames: Angled palate scissors, angular palate scissors, Trusler-Dean scissors

Uses: Dissection of the palate or oropharyngeal mucosa during palatoplasty, pharyngoplasty, and other oropharyngeal procedures.

Description: Scissors with a fulcrum (hinge) relatively close to their tines to allow for fine dissection. The tines are angled and may have a curve, whereas the shafts of the scissors may be straight (first image) or curved opposite to the tines to create an S-shape (last two images, which depict opposing sides of the same scissor).

Dimensions: 17 cm long

Tips and Pitfalls: These scissors come with a variety of tine angulations and shaft curves. Be sure to examine which are available to you and select the shape that is most ergonomic for the desired application. Be aware of the curve of the scissors and use them to your advantage.

Hockey Stick Elevator

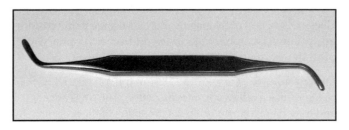

Aliases and Nicknames: Hockey stick (note that this instrument's name and nickname may also refer to other elevators of a grossly similar appearance)

Uses: Elevating mucoperiosteal flaps of the hard palate and bony alveolus in cleft repair.

Description: Double-ended elevator. Each end has a slightly curved, rounded tip, with opposite curvature on each end. One end is right sided and the other end is left sided.

Dimensions: 19 cm long

Tips and Pitfalls: Stay in a subperiosteal plane and avoid tearing the flap by keeping the tip of the elevator on bone throughout your motions. You should feel the tip of the elevator scraping gently against bone throughout your motion.

Double-Ended Palate Elevator

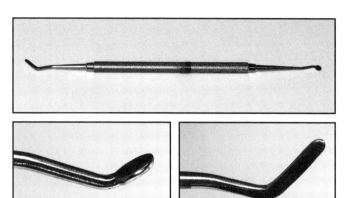

Uses: Elevating mucoperiosteal flaps off of the hard palate and bony alveolus in cleft repair.

Description: Double-ended elevator. One end has a flat, rounded tip, while the other has a longer, narrower tip with a rounded end.

Dimensions: 19 cm long

Tips and Pitfalls: Stay in a subperiosteal plane and avoid tearing the flap by keeping the tip of the elevator on bone throughout your motions. You should feel the tip of the elevator scraping gently against bone throughout your motion.

Mitchell Trimmer

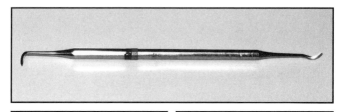

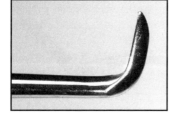
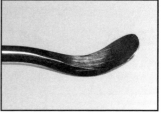

Aliases and Nicknames: Double-ended palate elevator

Uses: Elevating nasal floor mucosal flaps in cleft repair.

Description: Double-ended elevator. One end is sickle-shaped; the other is curved and rounded.

Dimensions: 16 cm long

Tips and Pitfalls: Avoid tearing the mucosal flaps by using gentle, controlled movements. The sickle-shaped end may be useful in starting your elevation, whereas the rounded end allows deeper dissection with less risk of tearing the flap.

Salyer Cleft Palate Elevator, 90°

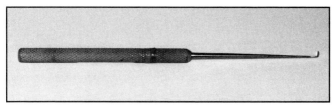

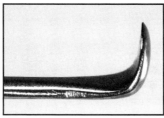

Uses: Used to define and begin elevating flaps at the cleft margins during cleft repair.

Description: Narrow, knurled handle, narrow neck, and 90° angled, rounded tip.

Dimensions: 18 cm long

Tips and Pitfalls: After incising the margins of the cleft, use this instrument to begin gently separating the edges of the nasal and oral flaps.

Single-Ended Palate Elevator, 90°

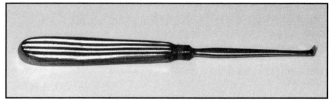

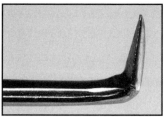

Uses: Used to define and begin elevating flaps at the cleft margins during cleft repair.

Description: Robust, grooved handle, narrow neck, and 90° angled, triangular pointed tip.

Dimensions: 16 cm long

Tips and Pitfalls: After incising the margins of the cleft, use this instrument to begin gently separating the edges of the nasal and palatal flaps.

Single-Ended Palate Elevator, Hooked

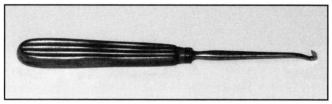

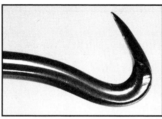

Uses: Used to define and begin elevating flaps at the cleft margins during cleft repair.

Description: Robust, grooved handle, narrow neck, and hooked, pointed tip.

Dimensions: 15 cm long

Tips and Pitfalls: After incising the margins of the cleft, use this instrument to begin gently separating the edges of the nasal and palatal flaps. The sharp curvature may be beneficial at the posterior edges of the cleft.

Grooved Director

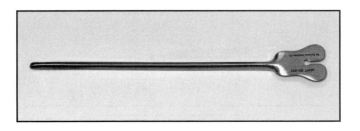

Aliases and Nicknames: Mickey Mouse

Uses: Lingual frenulectomy.

Description: Narrow handle/shaft with a flat, bilobed end that has a groove in its center.

Dimensions: 15 cm long

Tips and Pitfalls: Retract the tongue superiorly to expose the lingual frenulum, then insert the groove of this instrument around the frenulum. Superior retraction of the tongue with the instrument maintains exposure and access to the frenulum, which is then incised with scissors.

Pediatric Airway and Endoscopic Instruments

Fiber-Optic Light Carrier

See pp. 173–174

Light Clip

See pp. 175–176.

Pediatric Lindholm Laryngoscope

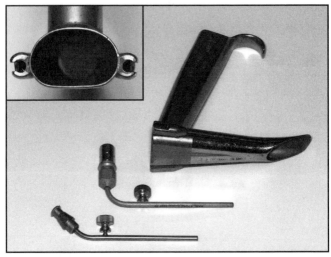

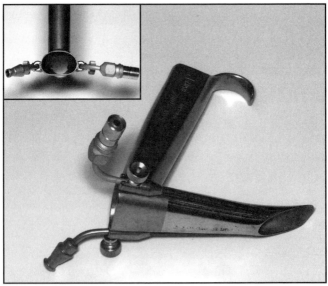

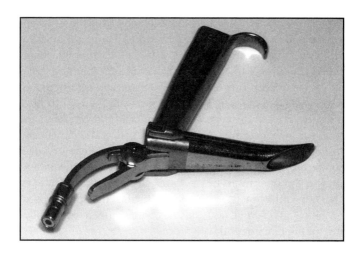

Note: For adult Lindholm laryngoscope, see pp. 158–159.

Aliases and Nicknames: Lindholm, Benjamin-Lindholm (neonatal size)

Uses: Direct laryngoscopy with or without microscope, telescope, laser or other endoscopic instruments.

Description: Angled handle with curved hook at its superior end. Body (blade) of laryngoscope is widest at the handle side and tapers to a narrow waist after which it flares out again. Tip has an upcurving, rounded prominence on its superior aspect. Lumen of laryngoscope is entirely enclosed, preventing obstruction of the surgeon's view by prolapsing tissue. One port on each side of the body holds a suction attachment or a fiberoptic light carrier (first and second images above with insets). May alternatively be used with a flat fiber-optic light clip that clips on to the inferior portion of body (bottom image above). Available in pediatric and neonatal sizes.

Dimensions: 9.5 cm long (neonatal size), 11 cm long (pediatric size)

Tips and Pitfalls: The Lindholm is a good first-choice laryngoscope for most pediatric applications. The wide opening allows plenty of working space, while the narrow waist and flared tip allow a fulcrum and working space for the distal ends of endoscopic instruments. The flared tip is designed to sit in the vallecula. The two side ports can be used to hold a light carrier and oxygen or suction without reducing the surgeon's working area. Note that the suction attachment can be kept on suction to clear smoke from laser or cautery, or it can be attached to an oxygen source to oxygenate the patient during the operation. In the latter case, be sure to put the "suction" attachment on the side of the laryngoscope closest to the oxygen source (eg, anesthesia machine) to avoid having tubing cross over the patient.

To perform endoscopic procedures during which two hands are needed for working, the laryngoscope is suspended and secured (see pp. 171–172). Note that the Lindholm is not an ideal intubating laryngoscope, as the endotracheal tube must be passed through the circumferential lumen of the scope. Removing the laryngoscope over the endotracheal tube is then difficult to achieve without extubating the patient.

Parsons Laryngoscope

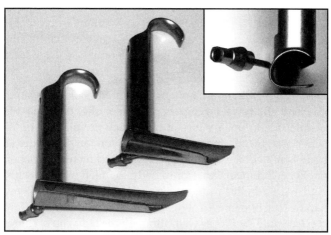

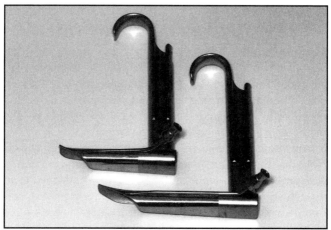

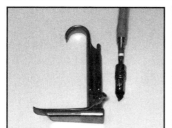
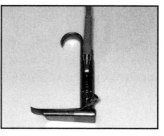

Aliases and Nicknames: Parsons, Benjamin-Parsons (neonatal size)

Uses: Direct laryngoscopy with or without microscope, telescope, laser, or other endoscopic instruments. Unlike the Lindholm laryngoscope, this instrument can be used to intubate with a small endotracheal tube if necessary.

Description: Straight handle with curved hook at its superior end. Body of laryngoscope tapers slightly from the handle side to tip. Tip has an upcurving prominence on its superior aspect. Lumen of body is open on the right side (ie, body is not circumferential). Built-in attachment for suction or oxygen tubing on left side of body. Requires a special light cord with a built-in prism that is inserted into the hollow handle (last two images above). May be used with a flat light clip (see pp. 175–176) as well, although the light clip occludes much of the lumen. Available in several sizes.

Dimensions: 9–11 cm long

Tips and Pitfalls: The Parsons is a good second choice in situations where the Lindholm fails to provide adequate visualization. The majority of the lumen is enclosed to prevent obstruction by prolapsing tissue, and the right-sided opening provides the right-handed surgeon greater working space to manipulate instruments through the laryngoscope. For these reasons, some surgeons use the Parsons as their first choice. Note that the suction attachment can be kept on suction to clear smoke from laser or cautery, or it can be attached to an oxygen source to oxygenate the patient during the operation. This scope is designed to be passed lateral to the tongue along the pharyngeal wall, rather than sweeping the tongue in the traditional manner. If the Parsons is used for intubation, the endotracheal tube can be passed through the right-sided opening in the lumen before the scope is removed. This laryngoscope can also be suspended (see pp. 171–172), allowing the surgeon to perform endolaryngeal surgery with two hands.

Rigid Bronchoscope

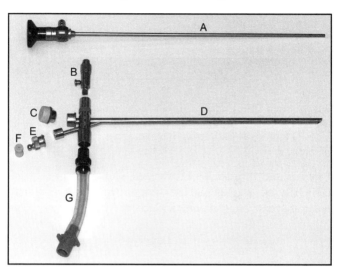

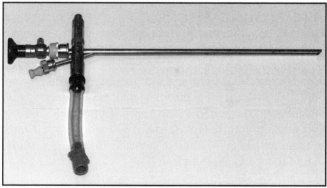

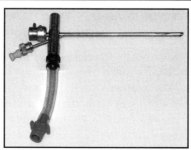

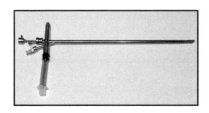

Aliases and Nicknames: Rigid bronch

Uses: Diagnostic and operative visualization of the subglottic airway.

Description: A multipart instrument with a long metal shaft (*D* in first image, unassembled). The proximal end of the shaft has transverse attachments that accept a light carrier prism (*B*) and ventilation tubing (*G*) as well as a central instrument port (*C* indicates its rubber diaphragm attachment) and a suction port (*E* and *F* indicate suction port attachments). The distal end of the shaft has three holes on each side and a beveled tip. Often used with a Hopkins telescope (*A*; see also pp. 127–129), or, alternatively, endoscopic foreign body forceps as discussed later in this chapter.

Images above depict the pediatric size (second image, note the rubber diaphragm attachment over the central port with inserted Hopkins telescope), neonatal size (third image, note the metal locking attachment over the central port without an inserted telescope), and adolescent (fourth image, note the metal "bridge" attachment over the central port without an inserted telescope).

Dimensions: Several sizes are available that vary in both diameter and length. Includes neonatal (including 2.5 mm, 3.0, 3.5, 4.0), pediatric (including 3.5, 4.0, 5.0), and adolescent sizes.

Tips and Pitfalls: The ability to assemble a bronchoscopic setup quickly and correctly is important, particularly in emergency situations in which a rigid bronchoscope may be your best option for airway control. Study the assembly instructions below and practice in nonemergent situations.

Note that for children beyond infancy, a 4.0 bronchoscope is usually a good first size to try. The 3.5 is also the smallest scope that will admit the optical foreign body forceps described later. In addition to the scope itself, you should have a Miller intubating laryngoscope (obtain from anesthesia), a 0° Hopkins telescope, appropriate suction, and a light source and light cord ready. Be sure to test your telescope and suction beforehand to ensure they are functional and the correct length for your bronchoscope.

When inserting the bronchoscope, use a Miller laryngoscope in the left hand to expose the glottis. At the glottis, rotate the bronchoscope so that the bevel faces laterally, and its narrow end can separate the vocal folds. Once you have engaged the subglottis, remove the laryngoscope, and advance the bronchoscope under telescopic (endoscopic) visualization. In doing so, hold the telescope and proximal end of the bronchoscope in one hand while you use the thumb and fingers of the other hand to protect the lips, teeth, and palate. To access each mainstem bronchus, gently turn the patient's head to the contralateral side. The side holes near the end of the scope allow ventilation of the contralateral lung while the scope is in a mainstem bronchus.

Assembly of the Bronchoscope:

Note: Setup applies to many adult rigid bronchoscopes as well.

1. Ensure that you have selected a bronchoscope (*D* in first image), not an esophagoscope.
2. Insert the light carrier prism (*B*) into the opening of the transverse metal tube at the proximal end of the bronchoscope. Insert until the first "click"; if you go any farther, the carrier will block the lumen of the bronchoscope, interfering with placement of the telescope. For modern applications, it is there only to prevent air escape from the system, not to actually carry light, as visualization will be performed using an illuminated Hopkins telescope.

3. Attach the ventilator circuit adapter tubing (*G*) to the bottom opening of the transverse metal tube. Only one end of the adapter will fit.

4. Assemble the rubber diaphragm attachment (*C*, assembled) by placing the rubber diaphragm over the flange of the metal adapter component. Then connect the metal component to the central port of the bronchoscope. Use of the rubber diaphragm allows easy transition from the telescope to other optical instruments (eg, endoscopic foreign body forceps) and suction. It also allows an airtight seal to form around these inserted instruments when providing positive pressure ventilation through the bronchoscope. (An alternative to the rubber diaphragm is a metal locking mechanism, which is pictured in the neonatal broncho-scope in the third image. The adolescent bronchoscope uses a special type of "bridge" adapter that is pictured in the fourth image.)

5. Slide a suction adapter (*E*) onto the diagonally oriented suction port at the proximal end of the scope. This port will have an off-center round opening. The adapter has a "0" that lines up with a "0" on the suction port. Once in place, slide the small rubber suction diaphragm (*F*) over the nipple on the adapter.

6. Last, place the desired type of telescope (eg, *A*) through the central port of the bronchoscope. The assembled bronchoscopic setup appears in the second image.

Rigid Esophagoscope

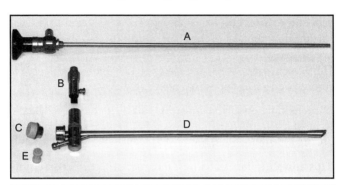

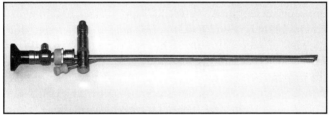

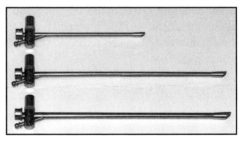

Note: For adult esophagoscope see p. 184.

Uses: Diagnostic and operative visualization of the esophagus.

Description: A multipart instrument with a long metal shaft (*D* in first image, unassembled). The proximal end of the shaft has a transverse attachment that accepts a light carrier prism (*B*) as well as a central instrument port (*C* indicates its rubber diaphragm attachment) and a suction port (*E* indicates suction port attachment). Unlike the bronchoscope, the shaft contains no ventilating ports and is cross-sectionally oval-shaped instead of circular. Also unlike the broncho-scope, the distal end has a slightly flared beveled tip that is thicker than the rest of the shaft. Study the assembly images above to learn these parts in more detail. May be used with Hopkins telescopes (*A*; see also pp. 127–128) or endoscopic foreign body telescopes (see next entry).

Dimensions: Available in various sizes, including #2 (19 cm long; at top in third image above), #3 (30 cm long; in middle), and #4 (30 cm long; on bottom).

Tips and Pitfalls: As with bronchoscopes, correct assembly is important. Be sure to have telescopes and suctions of the appropriate length. A "velvet-tip" suction (see p. 185) with a closed, blunt end and a side hole is a good choice to reduce the risk of mucosal injury when suctioning blindly. When inserting and advancing an esophagoscope, one hand holds the proximal end to rotate and steer the scope. The index and middle fingers of the other hand rest against the palate and upper teeth to protect them and provide a platform along which the scope slides. The thumb of that hand supports and advances the scope. In this manner, the scope can be advanced with minimal pressure, reducing the risk of muco-sal injury or perforation.

Assembly of the Esophagoscope:

1. Ensure that you have picked up an esophagoscope (*D* in first image), not a bronchoscope.
2. Insert the light carrier prism (*B*) into the top opening of the transverse metal tube at the proximal end of the esophagoscope. If you will be using a telescope or any instruments, insert only until the first "click"; if you go any farther, the carrier will block the lumen of the esophagoscope, interfering with placement of the telescope.
3. Assemble the rubber diaphragm attachment (*C*, assembled) by placing the rubber diaphragm over the flange of the metal adapter component. Then

connect the metal component to the central port of the esophagoscope. Use of the rubber diaphragm allows easy transition from the telescope to other optical instruments (eg, endoscopic foreign body forceps) and suction.

4. Slide the small rubber suction diaphragm (*E*) over the nipple on the suction port.

5. Last, place the desired type of telescope (eg, *A*) through the central port of the esophagoscope. The assembled esophagoscopic setup appears in the second image.

Endoscopic Foreign Body Forceps

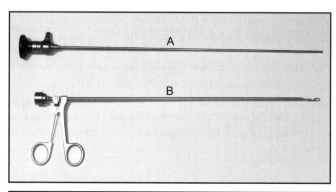

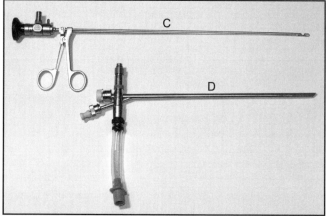

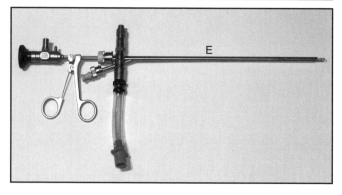

Aliases and Nicknames: Optical foreign body forceps, optical forceps

Uses: Endoscopic extraction of foreign material from the large airways or esophagus.

Description: A multipart instrument (*C*, assembled) designed to fit through a rigid bronchoscope (*D*) or rigid esophagoscope (not pictured). Parts include a thin rigid Hopkins telescope (*A*; see also 127–128) that locks into a hollow lumen grasping forceps (*B*). Forceps come in various shapes, most commonly "peanut forceps" with rounded, loop-like ends, and "coin forceps" with flat, alligator-like jaws.

Dimensions: The hollow lumen forceps (*B*) and associated thin rigid Hopkins telescopes (*A*) are available in pediatric and adolescent sizes. The two are not cross-compatible.

Tips and Pitfalls: The 3.5 bronchoscope is the smallest that will admit the endoscopic foreign body forceps. It is useful to set up the forceps with the tip shape you think most likely to be effective but to have other forceps available on your table as backup options. It also is wise to have a small (4 or 6 French) soft suction catheter available, as this can be threaded through the suction port of the bronchoscope or esophagoscope to clear the surgeon's view through the telescope. As with other rigid scopes, correct assembly is important. See below.

Assembly and Use of the Endoscopic Foreign Body Forceps:

1. Insert the thin Hopkins telescope (*A*) into the proximal end of the forceps (*B*). Once it is fully inserted, rotate the ring on the proximal end of the forceps to lock the telescope into the handles of the forceps. The light cord attachment should be positioned 180° from the forceps' handles to allow manipulation of the forceps.
2. Assemble your rigid bronchoscope (*D*) or esophagoscope (not pictured) separately as described in the previous entries.

3. Direct bronchoscopy or esophagoscopy is next performed using a wider diameter Hopkins telescope (which has superior optics; not pictured). Once the foreign body is identified the wider Hopkins telescope is removed.

4. Next, slide the assembled endoscopic foreign body forceps (C) through the rubber diaphragm into the instrument port of the bronchoscope (D) or esophagoscope (not pictured). The complete setup is pictured above (E, with bronchoscope). Take care to leave some space between the handles of the forceps and the proximal end of the bronchoscope or esophagoscope.

5. Secure the bronchoscope (or esophagoscope) in one hand and use the other hand to move the endoscopic foreign body forceps in and out of the bronchoscope (or esophagoscope) as needed. In addition to controlling the bronchoscope (or esophagoscope), the same hand can also be used to manipulate the patient's head and neck.

6. Once the foreign body is appropriately visualized, grasp and remove from patient. It is often safer to remove the entire assembly (eg, with bronchoscope or esophagoscope) from the patient in one unit, particularly if the foreign body will not fit through the lumen of the bronchoscope (or esophagoscope).

Myringotomy

Myringotomy Knife

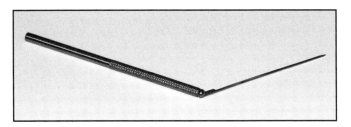

Aliases and Nicknames: Myringotomy blade

Uses: Incising the tympanic membrane for myringotomy or ear tube placement.

Description: Straight handle with straight blade; obtuse angle between handle and blade. Blade has a pointed tip, which is its cutting portion. Blade and handle may be a single unit, or handle may be reusable and accept disposable blades as shown in the image. Available in several varieties, including the interchangeable Beaver blade shown here.

Dimensions: 16 cm long

Tips and Pitfalls: The instrument should be controlled with your thumb, middle, and index fingers. Your fingers should approach the instrument at the obtuse angle between handle and blade. The base of the blade will sit near your index finger and thumb while the blade extends toward your 5th finger just in front of your fingertips. By holding the blade thus, you will be able to stabilize your hand while inserting the blade into the ear speculum or ear canal. As you insert the blade, be mindful of its sharp tip, which can scratch the ear canal and cause bleeding, and may obscure your view. When incising the tympanic membrane, gently insert the blade through the membrane. Avoid poking the blade tip into the underlying mucosa of the middle ear's medial wall, as this will also bleed.

Note: Refer to Chapter 2 for other instruments used during myringotomy (eg, aural specula, alligator forceps, Rosen needle, Frazier/Baron suctions, cerumen curettes).

CHAPTER

Facial Plastic and Reconstructive Surgery

**Prabhat K. Bhama, Kris S. Moe, and
Amit D. Bhrany**

CONTENTS

Stitch Scissors, Curved
Trusler-Dean Scissors
Long Metzenbaum Scissors

Elevators and Bone/Cartilage Instruments
Mead Mallet
#9 Molt Periosteal Elevator
Rowe Maxillary Disimpaction Forceps
Jansen-Middleton Septum Forceps
Beyer Bone Rongeur
Ruskin Rongeur
Gillies Bone and Zygomatic Hook
Dingman Zygoma Elevator
Boies Nasal Fracture Elevator
Langenbeck Elevator (Narrow Tip)
Langenbeck Elevator (Spatulated Tip)
Cushing Wide Sharp Elevator (Convex Edge)
Sheehan Nasal Osteotome
Aufricht Glabellar Rasp
Parkes Rasp
Fomon Rasp
Asch Septal-Reduction Forceps
Freer Dissector
McKenty Septal Elevator
Pennington Septal Elevator
Cottle Septal Elevator
Gorney Suction Elevator
Lempert Periosteal Elevator
Joseph Periosteal Elevator
Freer Septal Knife
Ballenger Swivel Knife
Molt Curette
Anderson-Neivert Osteotome With Guard

Fine Needle Holders and Forceps
Petit-Point Olsen-Hegar Needle Holder
Webster Needle Holder
Petit-Point Ryder Needle Holder

Bayonet Needle Holder
Castroviejo Needle Holder
McCabe Facial Nerve Dissector
Paufique Universal Suturing Forceps
Bishop-Harmon Forceps

Oral Cavity Retractors and Mouth Gags
Sluder-Jansen Mouth Gag
Lip Retractor
Jennings Mouth Gag
Bite Block

Miscellaneous Instruments
Aston-Daniel Endoscope Sheath
Castroviejo Caliper
Jameson Caliper
Round Scalpel Handle
Lacrimal Probe
Castroviejo Double-Ended Lacrimal Dilator

Retractors

Joseph Hook (2 mm)

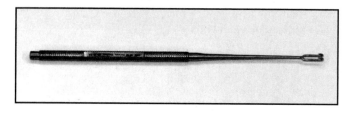

Aliases and Nicknames: Narrow double-prong hook

Uses: Retraction of skin and soft tissue.

Description: Narrow handle and shaft with sharp, narrow double-prong hooks.

Dimensions: 16 cm long

Tips and Pitfalls: Especially useful during rhinoplasty.

Fomon Nostril Elevator

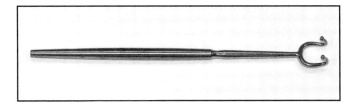

Aliases and Nicknames: Double-ball retractor

Uses: Retraction of nasal alae.

Description: Round, narrow handle with U-shaped distal end with curved tips terminating in balls.

Dimensions: 17 cm long

Rollet Retractor

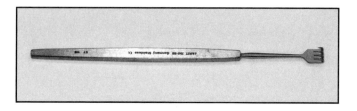

Uses: Retraction of skin.

Description: Narrow handle with 4-pronged sharp retractor.

Dimensions: 13 cm long

Tips and Pitfalls: More commonly used for oculoplastics procedures.

Aufricht Nasal Retractor

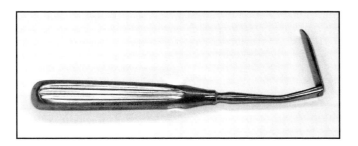

Uses: Cephalad retraction of nasal dorsal skin and soft tissue during open rhinoplasty.

Description: Large handle with bent shaft attached to retraction blade at 90°.

Dimensions: 19 cm long

Converse Blade Retractor

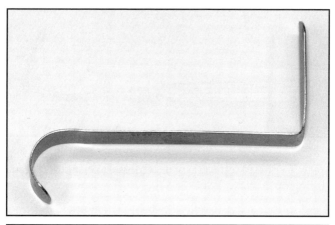

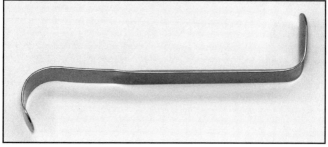

Uses: Retraction of soft tissue of the nose during open rhinoplasty.

Description: Flat midsection with one curved end and one 90° straight end.

Dimensions: 10 cm long, width varies

Tips and Pitfalls: The curved end can be handheld during retraction of the nasal soft tissue envelope with the straight blade. Alternatively, the straight blade can be clamped to a head wrap allowing the curved end to be used for cephalad retraction of nasal soft tissue, thus permitting hands-free use of the instrument.

Desmarres Lid Retractor

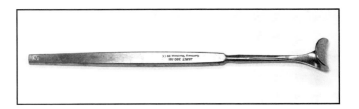

Aliases and Nicknames: Lid retractor

Uses: Retraction of eyelid. Typically used to retract lower eyelid during transconjunctival approach to the orbit or blepharoplasty.

Description: Slim handle with short shaft and curved distal end.

Dimensions: ~14 cm long (varies)

Ragnell Retractor

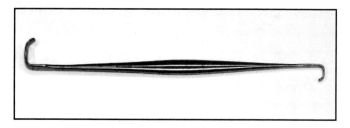

Aliases and Nicknames: Ragnell

Uses: Eyelid retraction.

Description: Double-ended retractor; each tip is more narrow than the tip of the Desmarres retractor.

Dimensions: 15 cm long

Tips and Pitfalls: Allows retraction of a narrower segment of lid farther than would be possible with the Desmarres retractor. Useful for confined regions.

Freeman Flap Rake Retractor

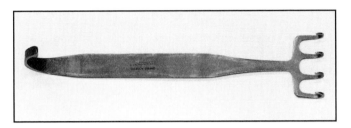

Aliases and Nicknames: Rake

Uses: Retraction of skin flaps during facelift, parotidectomy, or local flap reconstruction of the head and neck.

Description: The proximal end has single blunt hook for the surgeon's finger, and the distal end has four sharp hooks for skin retraction.

Dimensions: 10 cm long

Tips and Pitfalls: Use to pull the skin flap toward the surgeon to facilitate subcutaneous dissection, such as during facelift, parotidectomy, or local flap reconstruction.

Ferreira Facelift Retractor

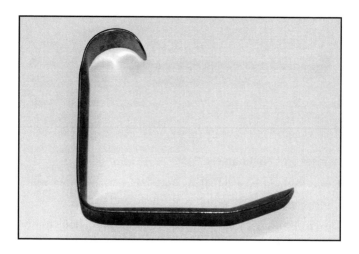

Uses: Retracting skin flap while elevating skin flap during facelift.

Description: Curved proximal end for surgeon's hands, gently angled at the distal end for retraction of skin flap.

Dimensions: Retracting end (bottom of image) is 10.5 cm long.

Scissors

Kaye-Freeman Rhytidectomy Scissors

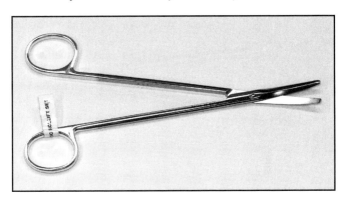

Aliases and Nicknames: Facelift scissors

Uses: Elevation of subcutaneous flaps during facelift, parotidectomy, or local flap reconstruction of the head and neck.

Description: Curved scissors with serrated blades and a ridge along the concave surface to help more easily dissect tissue.

Dimensions: 18 cm long

Tips and Pitfalls: Use with tips facing superficially when dissecting skin flaps. Ensuring that you can see the tips through the skin flap as you elevate helps indicate the appropriate depth of dissection. Push with the jaws slightly open to separate tissue in a gliding motion without needing to open and close the tips.

Castanares Rhytidectomy Scissors

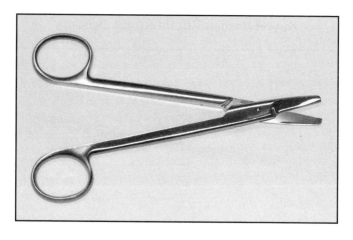

Uses: Separation of soft tissue during facelift.

Description: Scissors with short, stout, serrated blades.

Dimensions: 16 cm long

Tips and Pitfalls: Useful for dissecting vertical bands during facelift.

Westcott Scissors

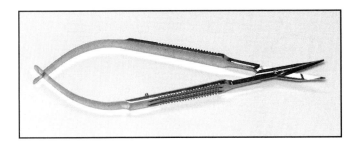

Aliases and Nicknames: Westcotts

Uses: Fine dissection of soft tissue, particularly in the peri-orbital region.

Description: Castroviejo-style nonlocking handle with sharp (or dull) tips.

Dimensions: ~12 cm long (varies)

Joseph Scissors, Curved

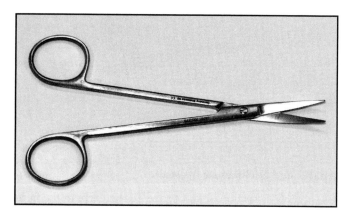

Aliases and Nicknames: Josephs

Uses: Cutting and dissecting soft tissue.

Description: Scissors with sharp tips; longer than iris scissors.

Dimensions: 14 cm long

Stitch Scissors, Curved

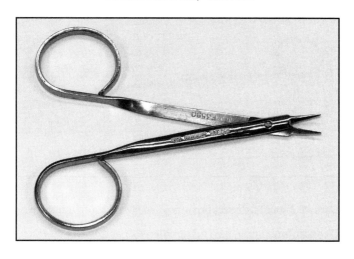

Aliases and Nicknames: Eye suture scissors, REEH stitch scissors, 3590 scissors, Weck scissors (slightly different models from different manufacturers)

Uses: Cutting fine sutures.

Description: Fine scissors with very distal hinge and fine tips.

Dimensions: 10 cm long

Tips and Pitfalls: Can be used for cutting suture, but also useful for fine dissection of soft tissue, such as elevating the soft tissue envelope off the lower lateral cartilages during open rhinoplasty.

Trusler-Dean Scissors

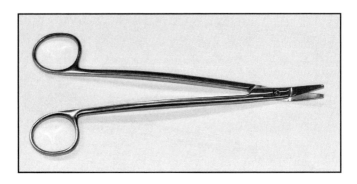

Uses: Submental dissection during facelift and submentoplasty.

Description: Long, curved handle with angulated tips.

Dimensions: 17 cm long

Tips and Pitfalls: Useful for direct excision of submental fat during neck lift.

Note: See also pp. 222–223 for their use in palate and oropharyngeal surgery.

Long Metzenbaum Scissors

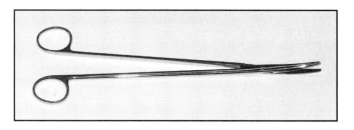

Aliases and Nicknames: Metz, long Metz

Uses: Dissection of soft tissue.

Description: Extremely long shanks (segment between finger rings and hinge) with slightly curved and blunt tips.

Dimensions: 29 cm long

Tips and Pitfalls: Orient tips parallel to important structures when dissecting. Similar to Kaye-Freeman rhytidectomy (facelift) scissors, they are useful for soft tissue dissection during elevation of subcutaneous flaps in facelift, parotidectomy, and local flap reconstruction. Also useful for neck dissection and separating fascial planes.

Elevators and Bone/Cartilage Instruments

Mead Mallet

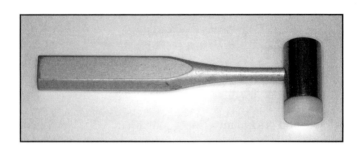

Aliases and Nicknames: Mallet, hammer

Uses: Used to strike osteotome or chisel during creation of osteotomies or sharp dissection of bone.

Description: Steel handle with weighted head. One side of the head is metal and the other side has a replaceable nylon cap.

Dimensions: 17 cm long

Tips and Pitfalls: Grasp mallet at handle and strike back end of osteotome or chisel by flexing at wrist only, not using your entire forearm. Allow the weight of mallet to provide the majority of force. Communicate with the surgeon holding the osteotome or chisel regarding how many times to strike the instrument.

#9 Molt Periosteal Elevator

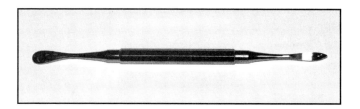

Aliases and Nicknames: #9

Uses: Elevation of periosteum from bone, eg, exposing the site of a fracture.

Description: Long, texturized shaft that acts as a handle with two ends: a pointed end with a subtle curve (on right in above image), and a rounded end with a subtle curve in the opposite direction (on left in above image). Both ends taper to a fine edge to enable elevation.

Dimensions: 18 cm long

Rowe Maxillary Disimpaction Forceps

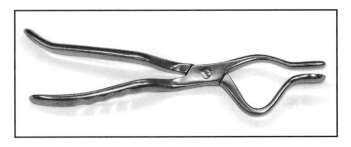

Aliases and Nicknames: Disimpaction forceps

Uses: To reduce midface/LeFort fractures. Also used to down-fracture the maxilla in LeFort I osteotomy.

Description: Side-specific forceps with a slightly curved blade (on top in above image) that is inserted into the nasal floor and a more acutely curved blade (on bottom in above image) placed underneath the palate.

Dimensions: 24 cm long

Tips and Pitfalls: Insert slightly curved blade into the nasal cavity and acutely bent blade into the oral cavity. The large bend in the lower blade accommodates the alveolus and protects the dentition of the maxilla. Allows for precise 3-D movement of fracture fragments.

Jansen-Middleton Septum Forceps

See p. 148.

Beyer Bone Rongeur

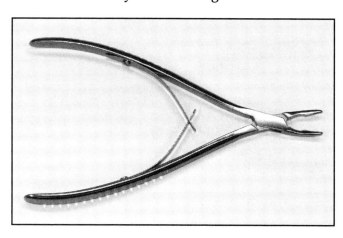

Aliases and Nicknames: Fine bone rongeur

Uses: Removal of bone.

Description: Tips have a fine/sharp surface to allow removal of bone.

Dimensions: 19 cm long

Tips and Pitfalls: Useful for removing bone off of maxillary crest and nasal spine during septoplasty. For removal of thick bone, use the Ruskin rongeur (see next entry).

Ruskin Rongeur

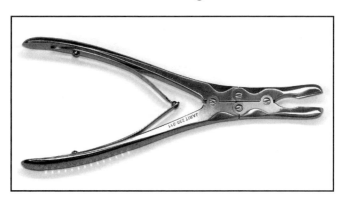

Aliases and Nicknames: Bone rongeur, heavy double-action rongeur

Uses: Removal of bone.

Description: Double-action mechanism with wide tips.

Dimensions: 19 cm long (varies)

Tips and Pitfalls: Useful for heavy, thick bone not amenable to removal with finer Beyer rongeur.

Gillies Bone and Zygomatic Hook

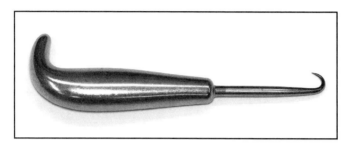

Aliases and Nicknames: Bone hook

Uses: Reduction of bony fractures requiring firm grasp of bone. Also useful for grasping medullary bone.

Description: Large handle with sharp, hooked tip.

Dimensions: 18 cm long

Tips and Pitfalls: Be careful to avoid applying too much pressure, which could fracture bone.

Dingman Zygoma Elevator

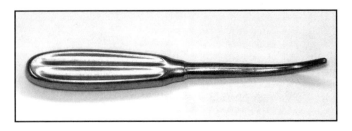

Aliases and Nicknames: Joker (note that the nickname joker also refers to an Adson periosteal elevator)

Uses: Elevation of depressed zygomatic arch fracture.

Description: Thick handle with curved, blunt tip.

Dimensions: 21 cm long

Tips and Pitfalls: When reducing zygomatic arch fracture, elevate the entire instrument as opposed to using a cantilever action.

Boies Nasal Fracture Elevator

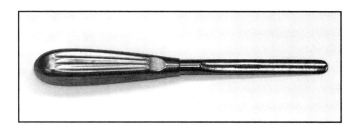

Aliases and Nicknames: Butter knife

Uses: Reduction of nasal fractures.

Description: Thick handle with straight, flattened blunt tip. Differs from *Goldman elevator,* which tapers in width as the instrument progresses distally.

Dimensions: 20 cm long

Tips and Pitfalls: Ensure that elevator is fully seated under nasal bones prior to reducing fracture. Can measure distance from ala to depressed nasal bone fragment and mark on the elevator. Elevate depressed side first, elevating entire nasal pyramid. Then repeat on other side to ensure straight nasal pyramid.

Langenbeck Elevator (Narrow Tip)

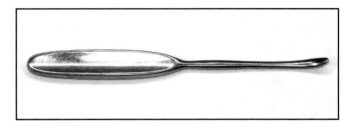

Aliases and Nicknames: Periosteal elevator

Uses: Elevation of periosteum from bone.

Description: Handle attached to narrow shaft with blunt, narrow, curved tip.

Dimensions: 21 cm long

Langenbeck Elevator (Spatulated Tip)

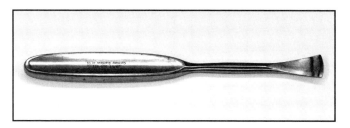

Aliases and Nicknames: Periosteal elevator

Uses: Elevation of periosteum from bone, including pericranium.

Description: Handle attached to narrow shaft with spatula-shaped sharp tip.

Dimensions: 20 cm long

Cushing Wide Sharp Elevator (Convex Edge)

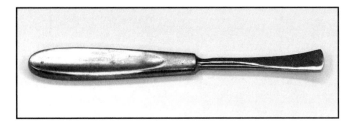

Uses: Elevation or dissection of soft tissue.

Description: Contains a spatula-shaped sharp tip (less sharp than a spatulated Langenbeck).

Dimensions: 19 cm long

Sheehan Nasal Osteotome

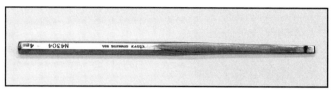

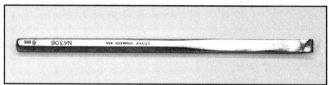

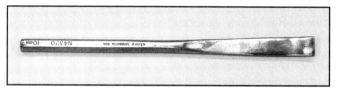

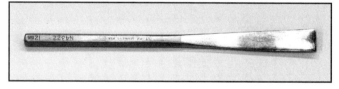

Aliases and Nicknames: Osteotome

Uses: Used with mallet for sharp dissection for removal of bone. Also used for nasal osteotomies for straightening the nasal dorsum.

Description: Narrow handle with flattened distal sharp spatulated tip.

Dimensions: ~16 cm long, width varies

Aufricht Glabellar Rasp

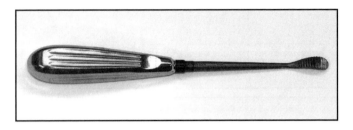

Aliases and Nicknames: Glabellar rasp

Uses: Removing bone at radix.

Description: Large handle. Tip is curved with transverse grooves on the convex surface designed for rasping.

Dimensions: 20 cm long

Parkes Rasp

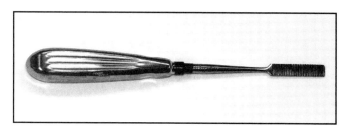

Aliases and Nicknames: Rasp

Uses: Contouring of nasal bone.

Description: Large handle. Tip is straight and rectangular with transverse grooves designed for rasping.

Dimensions: 20 cm long

Tips and Pitfalls: Removes bone with pulling motion.

Fomon Rasp

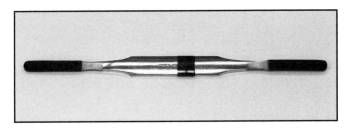

Aliases and Nicknames: Rasp

Uses: Contouring of nasal bones.

Description: Ends have a rough texture for rasping. Various types are available, with each instrument having a coarser and finer end. The finer end is higher in number.

Dimensions: 23 cm long

Tips and Pitfalls: Removes bone with both pushing and pulling motions.

Asch Septal-Reduction Forceps

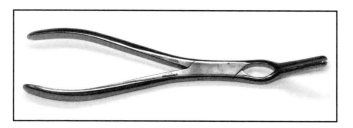

Aliases and Nicknames: Asch septal-straightening forceps, Asch forceps

Uses: Reduction of fractured nasal septum.

Description: Tines do not approximate completely, allowing for minimally traumatic manipulation of the septum.

Dimensions: 22 cm long

Tips and Pitfalls: Tips of the instrument may be directed inferiorly or superiorly along septum as needed.

Freer Dissector

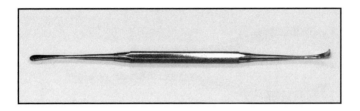

Aliases and Nicknames: Freer elevator, Freer

Uses: Blunt elevation of soft tissue, such as elevation of mucoperichondrium during septoplasty.

Description: Central handle with two curved tips for elevation of soft tissue. A *Freer suction dissector* is also available.

Dimensions: 18 cm long

McKenty Septal Elevator

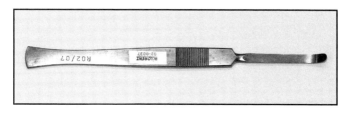

Uses: Elevating mucopericondrium from septal cartilage and bone.

Description: Flat handle with curved, sharp, rounded tip.

Dimensions: 15 cm long

Pennington Septal Elevator

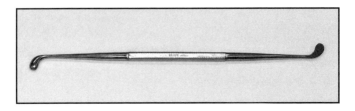

Aliases and Nicknames: Hockey stick elevator (note that this nickname may refer to other elevators of a grossly similar appearance)

Uses: Elevation of soft tissue, particularly retrograde dissection of mucoperichondrium from septal cartilage and bone.

Description: Straight central handle with two ends (tips) shaped like hockey sticks. One side of each tip is flat and the other side is curved.

Dimensions: 22 cm long

Tips and Pitfalls: Useful for dissection along maxillary crest to separate bands of mucoperiosteal flap from the crest.

Cottle Septal Elevator

See p. 130.

Gorney Suction Elevator

See p. 131.

Lempert Periosteal Elevator

See p. 78.

Joseph Perisoteal Elevator

See p. 79.

Freer Septal Knife

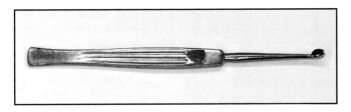

Aliases and Nicknames: D-knife

Uses: Incision of septal cartilage during septoplasty. Also useful for separating mucoperiosteom off maxillary crest.

Description: Thick handle with round shaft and sharp, D-shaped tip.

Dimensions: 16 cm long

Ballenger Swivel Knife

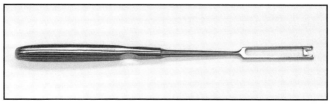

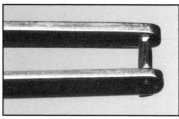

Aliases and Nicknames: Swivel knife

Uses: Incision of septal cartilage.

Description: Looks like a tuning fork with a blade on a pivot at the distal end that can rotate 360°.

Dimensions: 19–22 cm long (varies)

Molt Curette

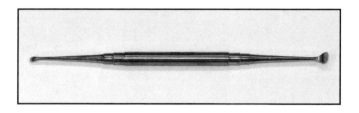

Aliases and Nicknames: Molt elevator, #2/4 Molt curette

Uses: Elevation of periosteum from bone.

Description: Rounded central handle with a rounded, curved tip at each end. One tip is slightly larger than the other. The tips are relatively sharp.

Dimensions: 19 cm long

Anderson-Neivert Osteotome With Guard

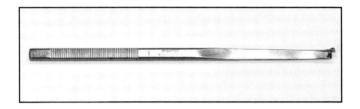

Aliases and Nicknames: Guarded osteotome

Uses: Cutting bone sharply.

Description: Thin, sharp tip with knob on one side that serves as a guard. The guard can be used to palpate the location of the instrument transcutaneously during osteotomy, and functions to maintain the osteotome on the surface of the bone.

Dimensions: 20 cm long

Tips and Pitfalls: When originally designed, the guarded end was intended to be placed on the mucosal side of the osteotomy to protect the mucosa from laceration. Now, the guarded end is more commonly placed on the cutaneous side to facilitate palpation of the osteotome's tip.

Fine Needle Holders and Forceps

Petit-Point Olsen-Hegar Needle Holder

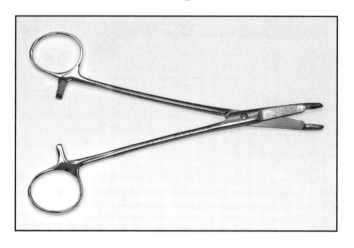

Uses: The combined needle holder and scissor allows the surgeon to drive needles and cut suture to avoid using an assistant or changing instruments.

Description: Ratcheted clamp mechanism. Fine needle holder (distal tip) with built-in scissor tines for cutting suture (just proximal to the tip).

Dimensions: 17 cm long

Tips and Pitfalls: Be careful not to accidentally cut the suture prematurely, particularly during a running stitch.

Webster Needle Holder

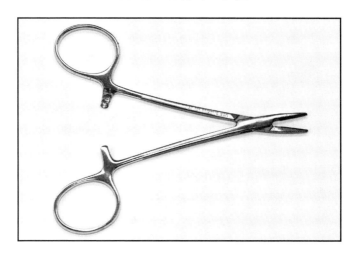

Aliases and Nicknames: Webster

Uses: Holding fine needles.

Description: Ratcheted clamp mechanism with short and fine design for holding small needles.

Dimensions: 12 cm long

Petit-Point Ryder Needle Holder

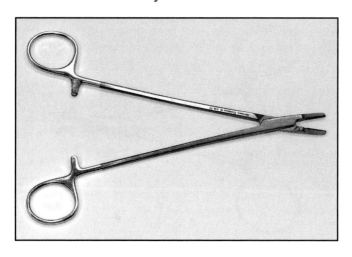

Aliases and Nicknames: Fine needle holder

Uses: Holding fine needles.

Description: Ratcheted clamp mechanism with long shank (segment between ratchet and hinge) and fine, narrow needle-holding tip.

Dimensions: 19 cm long

Tips and Pitfalls: Use with large needles may damage instrument jaws.

Bayonet Needle Holder

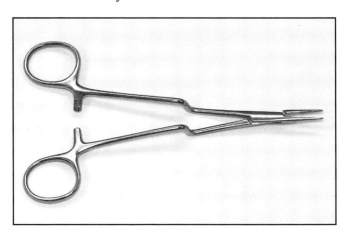

Uses: Suturing in a hole with narrow visualization (eg, the nasal cavity).

Description: Ratcheted clamp mechanism with bayonet design that offsets the tip from the handle.

Dimensions: 18 cm long

Tips and Pitfalls: Permits visualization of needle via a step-off (offset) in the handle. Ideal when working in a confined space.

Castroviejo Needle Holder

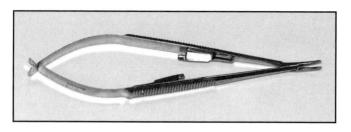

Aliases and Nicknames: Castros

Uses: Holding small needles, microsurgery.

Description: Microsurgical non-ring-handled design with locking handle (also available as nonlocking). Tips are very fine and may be curved or straight.

Dimensions: 14 cm long

Tips and Pitfalls: Commonly used in oculoplastic applications.

McCabe Facial Nerve Dissector

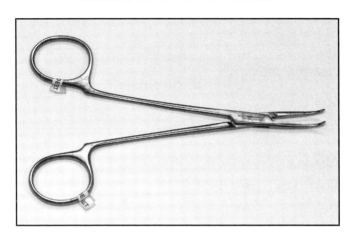

Aliases and Nicknames: McCabe

Uses: Elevation of soft tissue from facial nerve during parotid surgery.

Description: Ring handle without a ratchet mechanism, fine curved tips.

Dimensions: 14 cm long

Tips and Pitfalls: Insert parallel to nerve and gently lift the soft tissue off the nerve to expose to assistant for dividing. Avoid closing the tips once the tissue is elevated to prevent inadvertent crushing of the nerve.

Paufique Universal Suturing Forceps

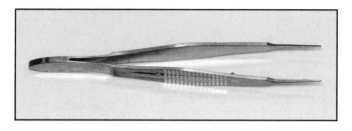

Aliases and Nicknames: Paufique

Uses: Handling soft tissue.

Description: Small, delicate forceps with fine teeth.

Dimensions: 9 cm long

Tips and Pitfalls: Often confused with the similar *0.5-mm Castroviejo suture forceps*. Handle tissue with care while using these forceps, as their sharp teeth can puncture and traumatize skin and soft tissue. Useful for fine tissue grasping.

Bishop-Harmon Forceps

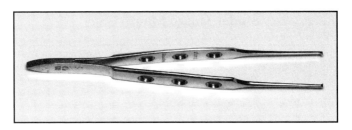

Aliases and Nicknames: Bishops

Uses: Handling soft tissue.

Description: Small, delicate forceps with fine teeth (similar designs are available without teeth). Grip area contains three holes on each side. Similar in design to Paufique forceps.

Dimensions: 9 cm long

Tips and Pitfalls: Handle tissue with care while using these, as the sharp teeth can puncture and traumatize skin and soft tissue. Useful for fine tissue grasping.

Oral Cavity Retractors and Mouth Gags

Sluder-Jansen Mouth Gag

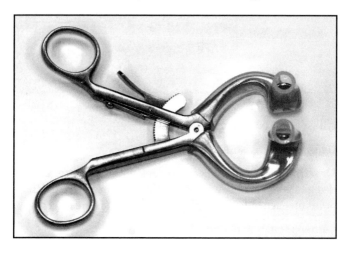

Aliases and Nicknames: Mouth gag, side-biting mouth prop

Uses: Retraction of mandible from maxilla to provide access to oral cavity.

Description: Ratcheted instrument with curved distal ends to accommodate dentition. Soft sheath over distal end to protect enamel.

Dimensions: 14 cm long

Tips and Pitfalls: Place at molars to avoid damage to dentition.

Lip Retractor

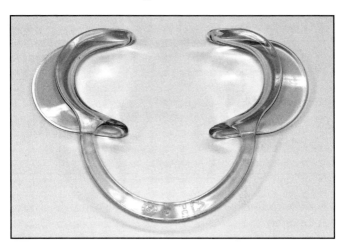

Aliases and Nicknames: Smile maker, cheek retractor

Uses: Retraction of lips for exposure of oral cavity.

Description: Made of plastic, retains memory for easy insertion into oral cavity.

Dimensions: 13 cm long

Tips and Pitfalls: Can be sutured to cheeks to prevent dislodging of retractor.

Jennings Mouth Gag

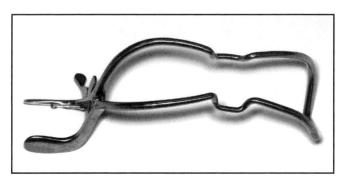

Uses: Retraction of mandible from maxilla to provide access to oral cavity.

Description: Large, ratcheting mouth gag.

Dimensions: 20 cm long

Tips and Pitfalls: Useful when access requirements prevent use of a bite block.

Bite Block

See p. 36.

Note: For other mouth gags (retractors), see pp. 209–214.

Miscellaneous Instruments

Aston-Daniel Endoscope Sheath

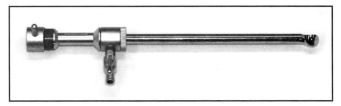

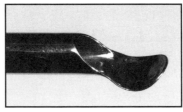

Uses: Visualization and illumination during dissection. The 30° endoscope (telescope) is placed into the sheath to shield the scope tip from surrounding tissue by increasing elevation of surrounding tissue during endoscopic brow lift.

Description: Sheath that accommodates the endoscope, which slides in and locks into place.

Dimensions: 4 mm diameter

Tips and Pitfalls: Sheath held with nondominant hand or by assistant during endoscopic brow lift. Avoid getting blood on the scope tip by elevating the skin of the incision as the scope is inserted.

Castroviejo Caliper

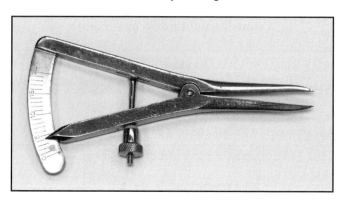

Aliases and Nicknames: Caliper

Uses: Distance measurements.

Description: Sharp, pointed tips with ruler-like device at opposite end. Thumb screw allows opening/closing of tips. Graded in millimeters.

Dimensions: 9 cm long

Jameson Caliper

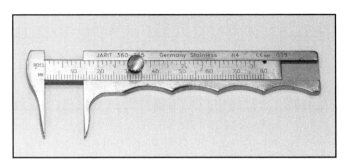

Aliases and Nicknames: Caliper

Uses: Distance measurements.

Description: Sliding caliper with locking screw. Graded in millimeters.

Dimensions: 10 cm long

Tips and Pitfalls: Allows measurement of larger distances than the Castroviejo caliper.

Round Scalpel Handle

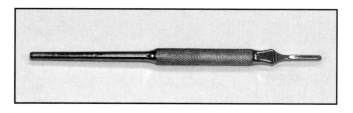

Uses: For curved incisions, or incisions that require rotation.

Description: Rounded, textured scalpel handle.

Dimensions: 16 cm long

Tips and Pitfalls: Increases ease of manipulation by permitting rotation between the fingertips, rather than requiring wrist movement such as with a standard scalpel handle.

Lacrimal Probe

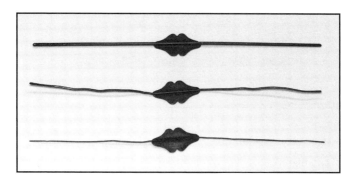

Uses: Probing of the lacrimal punctae or salivary ducts, retraction and protection of lacrimal canaliculi during trans-conjunctival procedures.

Description: Central handle with round probing ends at either side. Each end is a different gauge.

Dimensions: Varies

Tips and Pitfalls: Dilation is often better performed with a lacrimal dilator (see next entry) than with lacrimal probes.

Castroviejo Double-Ended Lacrimal Dilator

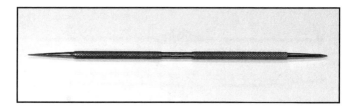

Aliases and Nicknames: Lacrimal dilator

Uses: Dilation of lacrimal ducts, other uses are similar to lacrimal probes.

Description: Central cylindrical handle with sharp tapered tips on both sides. One tip is sharper than the other.

Dimensions: 14 cm long

Index

Benjamin-Lindholm
 laryngoscope. *See*
 pediatric Lindholm
 laryngoscope.
Benjamin-Parsons
 laryngoscope. *See*
 Parsons laryngoscope.
Beyer bone rongeur, 271
bipolar cautery forceps, 50
Bishop-Harmon forceps, 299
bit. *See* drill bit (bur).
bite block, 36
blade, defined, xvi. *See also*
 scalpel blade.
Blitzer blade. *See* laryngeal
 sickle knife.
Boies nasal fracture elevator,
 275
bone hook. *See* Gillies bone
 and zygomatic hook.
bone/cartilage instruments
 for plastic and
 reconstructive surgery,
 268–291
bone rongeur. *See* Ruskin
 rongeur.
Bovie electrocautery, 5, 51–52
Brackmann suction, 72
bronchoscope, rigid, 237–240
Buckingham mirror
 large, 118
 small, 119
bur. *See* drill bit (bur).
butter knife. *See* Boies nasal
 fracture elevator.

C

caliper, 304–305
canal knife. *See* round knife.
cartilage instruments for
 plastic and reconstructive
surgery. *See* bone/
 cartilage instruments for
 plastic and reconstructive
 surgery.
carving block, 99
Castanares rhytidectomy
 scissors, 262
Castroviejo caliper, 304
Castroviejo double-ended
 lacrimal dilator, 308
Castroviejo needle holder,
 296
cautery. *See* Bovie
 electrocautery.
cerumen curette, 95
cerumen loop, 96
cheek retractor
 as nickname for University
  of Minnesota retractor, 35
 as nickname for lip
  retractor, 301
choanal curette, 217
claw. *See* electrode claw.
clip. *See* vascular clip applier.
cold knife. *See* Fischer knife.
converse blade retractor,
 256
Cottle septum elevator, 130
cricoid hook, 188
Crile forceps, 11
Crowe-Davis retractor, 212
Cummings retractor, 26
cup forceps
 laryngologic, 192
 otologic, 85–87
cup bayonet forceps, 91
curette, 92–96, 136, 149,
 215–217, 290
Cushing wide sharp elevator
 (convex edge), 278
cutting block. *See* carving
 block.

D

D-knife. *See* Freer septal
    knife.
Da Vinci robot EndoWrist
    instruments, 56–57
Deaver retractor, 28
DeBakey forceps, 5
debrider. *See* microdebrider.
Dedo laryngoscope, 163
dental mirror. *See* laryngeal
    mirror.
Desmarres lid retractor,
    257
Dingman retractor, 213–214
Dingman zygoma elevator,
    274
dilator, 189, 203–204
disimpaction forceps.
    See Rowe maxillary
    disimpaction forceps.
distal, defined, xvi
diverticuloscope. *See*
    Weerda distending
    diverticuloscope.
double-action, defined, xvi
double-ball retractor. *See*
    Fomon nostril elevator.
double-ended elevator, 199
double-ended palate elevator
    as nickname for Mitchell
        Trimmer, 226
    instrument of, 225
double-pronged hook, 39
downbiter, straight. *See*
    Kerrison rongeur,
    straight downbiting.
drill, 120–122
drill bit (bur), 120–122, 139
dual chamber light carrier,
    177
duckbill elevator, 81

E

ear cup forceps
    large, 85
    micro, 87
    mini, 86
ear loop. *See* cerumen loop.
ear speculum. *See* aural
    speculum.
electrode claw, 90
elevator
    as nickname for spatula,
        195
    group of instruments,
        78–81, 130–131, 195,
        198–199, 224–229, 253,
        269, 274–278, 284–286.
endoscope. *See* telescope.
endoscopic foreign body
    forceps, 244–246
EndoWrist instruments. *See*
    Da Vinci robot EndoWrist
    instruments.
esophageal dilator. *See*
    Jackson esophageal
    dilator.
esophagoscope accessories,
    185–186
esophagoscope, rigid
    adult, 184
    pediatric, 241–243
Essar suction irrigator, 77
eye suture scissors. *See* stitch
    scissors, curved.

F

facelift scissors. *See* Kaye-
    Freeman rhytidectomy
    scissors.
Farrior rasp. *See* oval window
    raspatory.